An Essay on Fevers

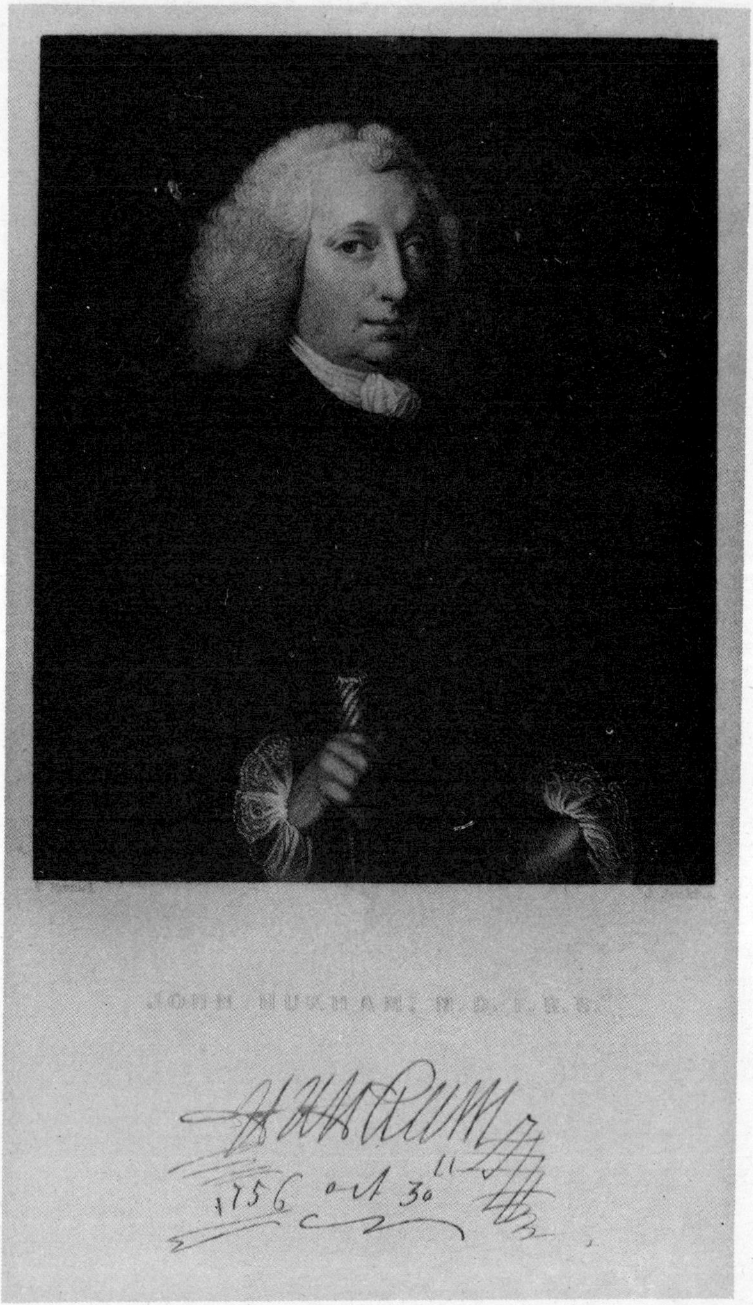

John Huxham (1692–1768)

John Huxham

An Essay on Fevers

Introduction by Saul Jarcho, M.D.

Science History Publications
U.S.A.

Originally published in 1757 (third edition) in London, England,
by J. Hinton. Reprinted with a new introduction by
Saul Jarcho, M.D.

Published in the United States of America
by Science History Publications/U.S.A.
a division of
Watson Publishing International
P.O. Box 493, Canton, MA 02021

The present study is one of a series of *Resources in Medical History*, selected in collaboration with the American Association for the History of Medicine, and funded under the Special Foreign Currency Program of the International Programs Branch, National Library of Medicine, Bethesda, Maryland

Library of Congress Cataloging-in-Publication Data

Huxham, John, 1692–1768.
An essay on fevers.

(Resources in medical history)
Reprint. Originally published: 3rd ed. London: J. Hinton, 1757.
Includes indexes.
1. Fever—Early works to 1800. I. Title. II. Series.
[DNLM: WZ 290 H986e 1757F]
RB129.H87 1986 616.07'2 86-11912
ISBN 0-88135-083-4

Typeset by Rekha Printers Pvt. Ltd., New Delhi and printed by
Amerind Publishing Co. Pvt. Ltd., New Delhi, India

Table of Contents

Introduction

In the middle decades of the eighteenth century Galenic doctrine still commanded widespread but not complete or uncontested allegiance in the world of medicine. New observations in anatomy, clinical medicine, and epidemiology had combined with Harveian and Baglivian physiology to reduce the dominance of ancient doctrinal systems but had not yet brought their reign to an end. At the same time new philosophical and taxonomic structures were being erected to accommodate new knowledge, while the value of ancient clinical observations did not lose recognition. Such, in brief, was the state of medical thought in the time of John Huxham, author of the classic work which is now being offered anew to medical and medicohistorical readers.

Of Huxham's biography[1] only a few facts need be recounted here. He was born in Devonshire in 1692, studied medicine with Boerhaave in Leyden in 1715, and obtained the doctoral degree at Rheims in 1717. Then he entered upon the practice of medicine at Plymouth. Activity as a practitioner did not deter him from intense study, and by the time of his death in 1768 he had gained distinction from both sources. The felicitous union of erudition and experience is evident in his writings.

Early in his career Huxham started to make meteorological and epidemiological observations. The statement which appears in the *Dictionary of National Biography*,[2] that his earliest observations on these subjects were published in the *Philosophical Transactions* for 1723, is not confirmed by examination of that periodical. It is true, however, that in a later book he refers to his previously recorded observations for the years 1724–1727. The *Index to the anatomical, medical, chirurgical, and physiological papers contained in the*

[1] N. Moore, "John Huxham" in *Dictionary of National Biography,* Compact edition (London: Oxford University Press, 1975), p. 1042.

[2] Ibid.

Transactions of the Royal Society of London (Westminster, 1814)[3] lists 14 articles contributed by Huxham during 1722–1762, but these deal mainly with observations in anatomy, surgery, and clinical rarities.

In 1739 Huxham issued his *Observationes de aëre et morbis epidemicis ab anno MDCCXXVIII ad finem anni MDCCXXXVII.*[4] This work reappeared in 1752 with a sequel containing observations made from 1738 to 1748. Other editions, in Latin and in English, were issued in 1758, 1759 and 1767.

Their titles immediately and correctly suggest a Hippocratic orientation. The texts open with prolegomena, sometimes extensive, on physical, meteorological, and physiological principles as then understood. The bulk of each volume consists of observations of wind and weather, pluviometric measurements, and the like, interspersed occasionally with brief essays on such subjects as icteric diseases and slow nervous fevers. Huxham appropriately remarked: "How very laborious such Works are, he only is capable of knowing, who has himself been concerned in them."

His famous essay on fevers, reproduced in the present volume,[5] is a direct continuation or culmination of the earlier *Observationes* and, indeed, uses some of the materials which are presented in those writings.

In the introduction Huxham points out that his earlier books did not afford sufficient opportunity for "particular Disquisitions on the Nature and Cure of the several Diseases."[6] The present volume therefore was designed to reveal his "Way of thinking and acting as to Fevers in general and those specified in particular," i.e. to discuss both theory and practice.

It was inevitable that Huxham's youthful study of Hippocrates should have led him to observe the relation between the weather of Plymouth and the diseases encountered in that city, nor is it very remarkable that an interest in Hippocrates should have led him to a discussion of the ancients in general, but at this point a surprise

[3]Royal Society of London. *Index to the anatomical, medical, chirurgical, and physiological papers contained in the Transactions of the Royal Society of London* (Westminster: Stace, 1814).

[4]London, Austen, 1739.

[5]John Huxham, *An essay on fevers.* 3d edition (reproduced in the present volume) (London: Hinton, 1757).

[6]Ibid., page xxv.

awaits the reader. Huxham explains that the great value of Hippocrates is that of having studied nature with great care and assiduity. The same, he says, is true of ancient poets and sculptors, who were the best copiers of nature. In other words, Huxham presents an esthetic doctrine of realism which originated in clinical writings and spread to include large areas of ancient art. It would be interesting to ascertain whether this philosophical sequence can be paralleled elsewhere in literature.

As to Galen, Huxham says laconically and politely that "the World would probably receive a judicious Abridgement of his Works with no small Satisfaction."[7] Indeed, throughout the present volume Galen is quoted much less often than Hippocrates, and the same order of preferences is in Huxham's earlier *Observationes.* However, we need not overlook the fact that Galen himself was a great admirer of Hippocrates, as is abundantly evident in the Hippocratic commentaries that are included in the *corpus Galenicum.* Moreover, Galenic influences are evident in many parts of the present volume, just as they are evident in most medical writings of the era, and also in nonmedical literature.

The opening chapter of Huxham's volume[8] reveals the difficulties experienced by our predecessors in their efforts to understand fever. Transmitting ancient doctrines supported in part by observation (interpreted correctly or not), Huxham says that running or other violent exercise will produce the febrile state. Exposure to cold moist air will suppress perspiration, increasing the quantity of the humors, and a feverish habit [condition] will ensue. A large ingestion of wine or spirits will increase the quantity of humors and will augment movement of the blood; this will produce a fever such as is known to occur after a drunken debauch. These conditions merely create a brief or ephemeral fever, quickly resolved by abstinence. But if the blood is greatly agitated and rarefied, it will be subjected to strong impetus, the blood vessels will be dilated, the globules will be forced into *serous arteries*[9] [lymphatics], and an inflammatory obstruction will be formed. When the thinnest part of the blood is dissipated, the remainder is thick. It is hampered in circulating and the residual serum comes to resemble jelly. This

[7]Ibid., page xxix.
[8]Ibid., p. 1.
[9]Ibid., p. 2.

process is the pathogenesis of "inflammatory fevers," such as peripneumony [pneumonia] and pleurisy. If the brain is affected, a "Phrenzy" is generated. All these conditions are worse if the blood previously had great strength in its fibers [fibrin] and if plethora was present.

The treatment, obviously, must consist of lessening the velocity, quantity, and acrimony of the blood by means of bleeding. When a patient is bled to the verge of fainting—the so-called bleeding *ad deliquium*—movement of the blood, says Huxham, almost ceases for a short time.[10]

Since it was also believed that the heat of fevers increased the acrimony of the body's animal salts and oils until the entire blood mass became putrid, and impacted matter at the ends of blood vessels and the beginning of serous vessels became more and more firmly lodged as a result of violent motion of the blood, delay in the application of bloodletting was dangerous. As a supplementary treatment thin, cooling, diluent liquids should be administered in order to overcome the continuous loss of lymph and serum and to keep the blood mass in a fluid state.

Acute inflammatory illnesses also were believed to have what we might designate nowadays as physicochemical characteristics. Febrile heat and friction, it was thought, cause animal salts to be "exalted" [intensified] and corrosive, and cause animal oils to become rancid and acid. When the serum of blood is jellied by heat and its oily component is increased, it becomes immiscible with water; hence something saponaceous, such as sugar [!] must be mixed with it. Sugared fruit juice is both acid and saponaceous [!][11] and hence is a diluent; presumably it prevents or resists thickening of the blood.

Another feature of fever is increased tension of fibers and vessels, an alteration which is caused by increased velocity, heat, and density of the blood. The tension is counteracted by diluents, especially when these are warm.

As might be expected, these tenets had implications which were important in therapeutics. Whereas gentle sweats were considered critical (in the Hippocratic sense) and could carry away a fever, profuse sweats were thought to be dangerous, especially at the onset

[10]Ibid., p. 3.
[11]Ibid., p. 5.

of pleurisy, pneumonia, or smallpox. The worst method of producing a sweat was by the use of certain alexipharmacal [antidotal] drugs or by smothering the patient in bedclothes. These "add Fewel to the Fire."[12] They increase the motion of the blood and hence the fever. Vesicants, to which Huxham usually but not invariably objected, might be undesirable because they throw acid salt into the blood and stimulate the fibers. After a bloodletting, emollient, cooling, laxative clysters are useful because they remove acrid bilious material which might otherwise be resorbed by the lacteals and enter the blood.

Huxham asserts that as increased velocity of the circulating humors will suffice to bring on a fever, all causes that increase this effect will act "in a compound ratio."[13] This remark suggests the influence of Newton and Bellini.

An important etiologic factor is diet. Huxham asserts that "the large Use of very salt and spiced Meats will raise a feverish Heat, even in the most healthy," but contrariwise, what are called slow or nervous fevers are generated by low, watery, unwholesome diet. Such fevers emanate from the *ultima vascula*—probably this means the ends of blood vessels—or the serous and lymphatic arteries, i.e. the lymphatics, and perhaps also from the points of origin of nerves.

Having set forth some of the fundamentals of pyretology, Huxham proceeds to consider the intermittent fevers.[14] Their procatarctic (predisposing) causes are a moist foggy atmosphere or continued rainy weather. These relax the fibers and obstruct perspiration. Consequently the blood becomes sluggish and may stagnate, obstructing the ends of blood vessels, as is shown by the observed fact that before a febrile paroxysm the patient becomes pale and his lips and fingertips may be livid. Similar appearances are produced by a cold bath.

If the circulatory sluggishness is great, and the patient's fibers are strong and tense, the fever will be high and the intermittent may turn into an acute continual fever. A hot regimen may convert an initial quotidian or tertian into an inflammatory fever, with "Phrenzy, Pleurisy, or Peripneumony;" this shows that the constitution of the bodily solids and fluids in some agues is not greatly

[12]Ibid., p. 6.
[13]Ibid., p. 9.
[14]Chap. 2, pp. 10–15.

different from that in inflammatory fevers. Experience gained in 1743 showed that catarrhal fever turned into quotidians and tertians, and observations made in 1744 showed that quotidian, semitertian, and tertian fevers might coexist with epidemic pleurisy and pneumonia.

Huxham inferred that when pleurisy, pneumonia, and inflammatory rheumatism are common in a cold dry spring and are succeeded by numerous intermittent fevers in the warmer months, this is because the heat of the new season has reduced the rigidity of fibers and has reduced the viscosity and density of the blood. To the twentieth-century physician this statement can only mean that vernal intermittents are milder than pleurisy and pneumonia. In consonance with such an interpretation Huxham remarks that "if you can turn a slow nervous fever [typhoid, mostly] into a regular Intermittent, you can soon cure your patient." In the contrary event, if the bodily solids had continued in a state of tension and the blood had continued to be viscid, inflammatory fevers would have continued to prevail if the weather were cold.

Like many another physician in his era, Huxham felt that excessively hasty administration of Peruvian bark[15] might turn a regular tertian fever into a semitertian or quotidian; hence he waited until at least four or five paroxysms had passed, especially in vernal agues. This widely held opinion illustrates the difficulty of ascertaining the character of a fever early in its course. Here Huxham had recourse to his own experience and also to experiments reported by Dr. Browne Langrish (d. 1759), a surgeon and experimental physiologist who had performed "a statical examination", in which he had attempted to measure the quantity of serum in the blood and the cohesiveness of the clot in intermitting, quotidian, and tertian fevers.

In his discussion Huxham mentioned not only these three categories but also used the ancient term *semitertian,*[16] which incidentally suggests a degree of nosologic or nomenclatural conservatism. He remarked, moreover, that "a regular Tertian is a Medium between an inflammatory and a slow nervous Fever." This translates approximately into the assertion that tertian malaria is physio-

[15]Page 12.
[16]Page 12.

logically intermediate between pneumonia or acute rheumatic fever and typhoid.

At this point in the exposition, in order to explain how the physician should act in spurring or bridling Nature during various fevers, Huxham intercalated into his essay a series of three special chapters[17] which deal with what might be called pathologic physiology. The first of the three discusses the flexibility and tension of the body, as illustrated by such conditions and occurrences as marasmus, dropsy, atrophy, and hemorrhage. The opinions and doctrines reflect ancient methodism and also the influence of Baglivi and of Huxham's teacher, Boerhaave. The second chapter[18] in the subseries discusses fluids, their density, viscosity, momentum, and friction, as well as plethora, sluggishness, and bad composition ("cacochymia"). The effect of disturbances in the solid and fluid departments is illustrated by Huxham's comment that "a weak watery Blood and a relaxed Habit of Body, where either considerably deviates from the Standard of Nature, . . . becomes a real disorder, and it is to be duly regarded in whatever concurring Disease happens."[19] This dictum Huxham amplified by a confident footnote which declares that ardent and inflammatory fevers result from excessive elasticity and rigidity of fibers and excessive density and viscosity of the blood, whereas slow and nervous fevers result from laxity of vessels and thinness of blood, while several diseases, especially those which are contagious, may manifest both groups of traits.

The third chapter in the subseries[20] discusses an extremely dangerous condition, viz. the dissolved and putrid state of the blood, held responsible for scurvy and for all other hemorrhagic disorders, including some kinds of snakebite and hemorrhagic smallpox. The hemorrhages in general are attributed to acrimonious humors which impair the *crasis* or mixed composition of the blood and corrode the termini of capillaries. The exposition of hemorrhage leads to a dramatic description of hemorrhagic smallpox and this leads in turn to an appalling report of a hemorrhagic fever, designated as a petechial fever (typhus? acute leukemia?).

[17]Chapters 3, 4, 5 (pp.15–38).

[18]Pp. 19–22.

[19]Page 22.

[20]Pp. 22–38.

These considerations lead to a separate brief chapter,[21] predominantly nosological and etiological rather than clinical, in which Huxham explains the difference between a slow nervous fever (mostly what we now call typhoid fever) and putrid malignant fever (mainly typhus). He declares that in putrid, malignant, and petechial fevers the blood is affected, whereas in slow nervous fevers the disease is situated principally in the lymphatic and nervous fluids. The former diseases commonly arise from contagion, the latter sometimes do. Cold, watery, and mucilaginous foods such as cucumber, melons, and some fruits, bring on slow nervous fevers without putrefaction, whereas hot, acrid, saline, and spicy foods cause putrid and malignant fevers.

The matters that have been discussed thus far constitute the first six chapters of Huxham's book and make up approximately one-third of its content. Arranged in an order that is hardly to be commended or imitated, they first consider inflammatory fevers and intermittent fevers, and then interrupt the series with a succession of digressions on solids, fluids, and dissolution of the blood. The procession of diseases resumes with chapters on "the slow nervous fever", the putrid, malignant, and petechial fevers, an essay on smallpox, and a three-chapter dissertation on pleurisy and pneumonia, which is in part a return to subjects discussed in the first chapter of the book. The unusual order in no wise impairs the notable clarity of the exposition, in both the theoretical and the clinical passages. The latter contain many treasures of exact observation, set forth succinctly, and these may be the reason for the prolonged popularity of the book.

Of the slow nervous fever,[22] which seems to be what we call typhoid fever, Huxham gives a minutely detailed description. For example, not content with mentioning headache, he specifies that the patient experiences obtuse pain and coldness in "the hinder part of the head" and heavy pain along the coronal suture. He is equally specific with regard to the location of the sweating. Any querulous reader who disputes these determinations is welcome to find a case of the disease and report the comparison to the present commentator. There is emphasis on the occurrence of deafness but no mention of bradycardia. Nothing is said about rose spots, but there is men-

[21] Pp. 38–40.
[22] Pp. 40–49.

tion of a miliary eruption. The description of the disease is clinical and there is no mention of the anatomical findings which would be diagnostically decisive.

Of the putrid, malignant, and petechial fevers, a group probably composed in part of what we now call typhus and in part of hemorrhagic diseases, Huxham says, not altogether logically, that they "Many times arise from mere antecedent Acrimony of the Blood, agitated by the supervening Fever [sic!], yet generally the pestilential and the petechial have their Origin from Contagion."[23] The contagion, he continues, acts in nearly the same manner as acrimony and will affect a vigorous and a weak constitution differently. In this context the word *contagion* can only signify a material object that is transmitted from one person to another. The alternative interpretation, viz. that contagion is a process of transmission, would confound efficient cause with material cause. Huxham's pronouncement, in addition, exemplifies his repeated and appropriate emphasis on human constitutional variation, an important factor in disease.

Huxham establishes clear clinical distinctions between the slow nervous fevers and the petechial pestilential ones. As before, he specifies the location of the headache (a prominent feature of typhus): he says it is bitemporal, supraorbital, and retroorbital.[24] He contrasts the throbbing of the carotid pulsation with the smallness or slowness of the radial pulse. He notes that prostration, weakness, and faintness occur despite the absence of any large evacuation. He carefully describes the appearance of the tongue, an organ which receives no more than perfunctory attention in present-day clinical practice, and he presents a detailed description of the petechiae and vibices. He also describes, briefly, other eruptions encountered during pestilential fevers; some of the lesions add to the evidence that diseases other than typhus were included in the same category.

In addition to presenting clinical descriptions Huxham explains in detail the reasons for bloodletting and its limitations. [25] Fever, he says, is an effort of nature to throw off offensive or morbid matter. Bloodletting performed at the onset of the illness reduces the fever and prevents it from producing inflammations "of the brain, lungs,

[23]Page 50.
[24]Page 50.
[25]Page 55.

and other vital parts," i.e. the complications most to be feared are pneumonia and "phrenzy." Bleeding does not remove the whole of the morbid material, since the latter is intimately mixed with the humors. In judging the progress of the illness and the effect of treatment, useful information could be obtained by observing the appearance of the blood that is drawn; this procedure can be regarded as the predecessor of modern laboratory tests, and similar considerations apply in part to observation of bodily discharges.

The phenomena observed during malignant and petechial fevers led Huxham to interesting inferences, based in part on the work of Giorgio Baglivi (1668–1707).[26] It was usual for the patients to have weakness, trembling, and dejection of spirits. It was inferred that the nerves and the [Galenic and pre-Galenic] animal spirits were affected by the contagious miasms which had caused the illness and became unable to actuate the muscle fibers and the blood vessels. This produced weakness and enfeebled "vibration" (pulsation?) of the vascular system. Consequently the blood coagulated in some places and dissolved in others. This inference was supported by observation: in persons who had died of plague the heart and auricles were found to be distended by grumous blood.

Huxham says that for many years he had used the Peruvian bark with success,[27] not only in intermittent and slow nervous fevers, but also in the putrid, pestilential, and petechial fevers, *especially during their decline* (italics added). The fact that in his statement about the bark Huxham mentions intermittent fevers before the other categories is possibly significant. It was surprising that he nowhere mentions Francesco Torti, whose classic work, first issued in 1712, had gone far to define the usefulness of the drug. Another surprise is that the chapter on putrid and pestilential fevers, and not the chapter on intermittent fevers, contains the recipe for Huxham's famous febrifugal tincture, an interesting mixture of Peruvian bark, the peel of Seville oranges, Virginia snakeroot, English crocus, Central American cochineal, and French brandy. The diverse origins of these components summarize a fascinating part of the history of pharmacy. Of the tincture the *New Edinburgh Dispensatory* of 1786 remarks (pp. 321–322) that "in some ill habits, particularly where the viscera and abdominal glands are obstructed, the bark, by itself, proves unsuccessful, if not injurious; whilst given in conjunction

[26] Pp. 56 ff.
[27] Page 65.

with 'stimulating' stomachics and deobstruents, it more rarely fails of due effect. Gentian and Virginian snakeroot are among the best additions for this purpose . . ." Toward the end of his chapter on putrid and pestilential diseases Huxham makes the sage remark that "the dietetic Part of Medicine is not so much studied as it deserves."

To confirm and extend the doctrines expounded in this chapter, Huxham, somewhat surprisingly, inserted an essay on smallpox.[28] This famous contribution is not a systematic treatise, but a somewhat random and nevertheless valuable collection of opinions and observations. Huxham, as always, was strongly impressed by the differences in the severity of the disease among different patients. He noticed that variolous pus often infected the skin of persons who had had the disease previously and produced a great number of pustules similar to those of smallpox, but without fever. This was a common occurrence among attendants.

Huxham emphasized the constitution of the air and the constitution of the patient, not only as an explanation of causes and symptoms but also as a determinant of treatment. He advocated bloodletting from the foot in the belief that it acts powerfully to draw the sickness from the head and breast [chest], two structures that should be guarded. This diversive procedure was still used in Huxham's time and can be viewed as an island of resistance to the Harveian doctrine of circulation. For similarly revulsive purposes Huxham would order warm baths for the feet and epispastics for the feet and wrists, and the patient's head would be shaved to keep it cool. Surprisingly, he advocated the use of vesicants in smallpox, but only in special circumstances. He opposed the use of emetics, since he believed that vomiting forces too much blood into the brain.

Another notable part of Huxham's book is a series of four chapters on pleurisy and peripneumonia.[29] Highly typical of the era is the first of the four, which explains the power of wind and weather in the etiology of these diseases. Huxham says that "persons of a very viscid State of the Blood and rigid Fibers are subject to inflammatory Disorders of all Kinds, in all Seasons; but some Constitutions of the Air. . . are not only more apt to produce this inflammatory Blood than others, but also dispose more to

[28] Pp. 67–88.
[29] Pp. 89–136.

Inflammations of particular Parts."[30] This pronouncement accounts for the fact that acute respiratory illnesses are commoner in some seasons of the year than in others, in some years more than others, and in some people more than others. Thus it simultaneously embraces the constitution of man and the constitution of the atomosphere.

Huxham's concepts of pathogenesis and taxonomy divide the pulmonary diseases here under consideration into three groups. The first, peripneumony, arises from violent inflammation of the lungs by a sizy [glutinous] dense blood which obstructs some of the pulmonary and bronchial arteries. This definition suggests that etiological significance was attributed to blood found post mortem in the arteries of the lungs. The second, *peripneumonia notha* (false or bastard pneumonia), allegedly caused by phlegm in the blood and lymph, probably refers to the modern bronchitis plus some cases of bronchopneumonia. The third, said to consist of a thin acrid defluxion, is probably what we now call pulmonary edema. Huxham wisely remarks that each particular disease in every individual patient, is to be considered by the attending physician not according to the nomenclature, but according to the nature, causes, and symptoms of that particular disease in that particular person.

* * *

Into the third edition (1757) of his *Essay on Fevers* Huxham inserted a chapter of twenty-four pages titled A Dissertation on the Malignant Ulcerous Sore-Throat.[31] This work, reprinted in subsequent editions and translations, has become famous and is regarded by some readers as a classic.

It opens with an admirably concise historical review, which recalls the important statements of Aretaeus and Aetius, and mentions indistinctly the observations of seventeenth-century Italian and Spanish authors as well as the recent contribution of Fothergill.

Huxham states that his experience with malignant sore throat abundantly confirmed his opinions about pestilential fevers, discussed in earlier pages of the present introduction. He had seen the disease first about 1750. His account starts with a detailed

[30] Page 91.
[31] Pp. 141–163.

account of weather and diseases month by month from the summer of 1751 through May of 1753.

The major descriptive passages in his exposition are, as usual in his writings, richly detailed. Among the features mentioned are:[32] acute onset; tendency for the symptoms to be most severe at night; foul breath, offensive *to the patient* as well as to attendants; anxiety, delirium, and insomnia; fever accompanied by relatively meager sweating; peculiarities of the voice, different from what is heard in quinsy; greater frequency of sneezing in children than in adults; excoriations and other lesions not only about the nose but also in many other parts of the body; and a tendency of cutaneous lesions to occur on the hands of attendants. The condition of the throat, mouth, and tongue is portrayed attentively. Paralysis is not mentioned.

Included with the clinical descriptions is a brief account of prognostic signs and of differential diagnosis.[33] Huxham considered the latter to be of special importance because he felt that bloodletting should be avoided in cases of malignant ulcerous sore throat, whereas the procedure might be permissible in other conditions which closely resemble it.

The clinical facts are accompanied by brief mention of the background, which is that of Plymouth, the famous seaport and naval base. The presence of French prisoners[34] and their physicians allowed Huxham to observe the tendency of the latter to use bloodletting in pestilential and other fevers with a freedom which he deemed excessive.

Despite the profusion of detail in Huxham's descriptions of malignant ulcerous sore-throat, it is by no means certain whether he was dealing solely with diphtheria or whether cases of scarlet fever and other pharyngeal infections were included in his sack of troubles. Similar misgivings were expressed by such distinguished physicians as Charles Creighton[35] and Arthur Bloomfield.[36] Indeed, the latter also had doubts concerning the subsequent descriptions

[32]Pp. 146 ff.

[33]Pp. 151 ff.

[34]Page 152.

[35]C. Creighton, *A history of epidemics* (Cambridge: Cambridge University Press, 1894), pp. 699–700.

[36]A. Bloomfield, *A bibliography of internal medicine: communicable diseases* (Chicago: University of Chicago Press, 1958), pp. 246–248.

by Bretonneau. These difficulties illustrate some of the limits of clinical diagnosis in the pre-bacteriological era.

* * *

The unmistakably Hippocratic tenor of Huxham's thinking and writing has been mentioned earlier in the present introductory analysis. The esteem that he felt for Hippocrates he also extended, for the same reasons, to other ancient clinicians, especially Aretaeus and Alexander of Tralles. He was less enthusiastic about Galen but did not undervalue the large number of excellent observations that occur in the midst of the Galenic plethora. The other authors whom Huxham mentions or quotes are spread across the Middle Ages and subsequent eras, from the time of Rhazes to that of Morton, Mead, and Friedrich Hoffmann. In this large series of major and minor authors Huxham found himself to be closest to Sydenham and to Boerhaave. Both Sydenham and Huxham centered their interests at the bedside and excelled in endlessly repeated minute observations, a method which is not infallible but which rarely fails to extend the scope of human knowledge. Both men saw or attempted to see close relations between weather and disease, and both were strongly inclined toward what we to-day call epidemiology. Sydenham disclaimed theory but could not escape it, while Huxham carried a large burden of theoretical concepts but was undistinguished as a theoretician.

Huxham mentions Willisian notions of fermentation and Willis' chemical principles (such as sulphur and salt) but he does not mention Willis. His thinking was much influenced by Baglivi's iatromechanical tendencies and especially by the Baglivian *De fibra motrice et morbosa.*[37] His treatise shows little inclination toward morbid anatomy, a subject which at that time was being advanced by the work of Morgagni and others. Surprisingly, he discusses the use of Peruvian bark but fails to mention Torti, and much of his work and thought was directed along epidemiological lines but he fails to mention Lancisi.

A great merit of Huxham's book resides in the clarity with which he explained his concepts and their application in treatment. Hence his treatise can be used as a textbook of eighteenth-century medicine, a subject which the lapse of two centuries has made

[37]Giorgio Baglivi, *Opera omnia* (Venice: Tomasinus, 1727), pp. 147–248.

increasingly difficult to understand. Here we are confronted by a paradox in that notably clear explanations are set forth in a book which is arranged on a confusing plan, discussed above. A further bit of confusion, almost a curiosum, is the fact that the principal discussion of Peruvian bark appears in the chapter on putrid malignant fevers, whereas the drug receives only relatively brief mention in the chapter on the intermittents.

It is reasonable to surmise that the usefulness of Huxham's *Essay* was due to the fact that over all the world and in all centuries fevers have been the commonest physical affliction of the human race. But the book was popular as well as useful, and this fact is demonstrated by the record of its publication. *The Short Title Catalogue of Eighteenth Century Printed Books in the National Library of Medicine* by Dr. John B. Blake (Bethesda, 1979, p. 227) lists ten London editions, which appeared during a period of three decades. It is not to be assumed that all of these were really new editions according to the standards of our time, since some are merely reprints of their immediate predecessors. For example, the first sentence of the author's preface reads "About ten Years ago I published . . ." This exordium persists unchanged at least as far as the sixth edition, issued in 1769, a year after Huxham's death. The third edition (1757) corrects an erratum noted in the second (1750); much more important, it adds the well-remembered Dissertation on the Malignant Ulcerous Sore-Throat.

Dr. Blake lists five Italian editions, issued in Naples and Venice, 1765–1786, and seven Paris editions, 1752–1776, with varied titles. In addition there are four editions issued in Leipzig 1764–1829, and titled *Opera physico-medica*, as well as extensive excerpts in encyclopedias. One of these appeared in Venice in 1836 in the seventh volume of the *Enciclopedia delle Scienze Mediche* (pp. 685–793) and is based on a French translation of 1765, which in turn is based on the third English edition (1757).

The historian will observe with interest that the major Italian and German editions are in Latin, whereas the British and French editions are in the respective vernaculars, and that no North American editions are on record.

It is pleasant to reflect that our long national dereliction will now be amended.

SAUL JARCHO, M.D.

AN

ESSAY

ON

FEVERS.

To which is now added,

A

DISSERTATION

ON THE

Malignant, Ulcerous SORE-THROAT.

The THIRD EDITION.

By JOHN HUXHAM, *M. D.*
Fellow of the *Royal College of Physicians* at *Edinburgh*,
and of the *Royal Society* at *London*.

LONDON:
Printed for J. HINTON, in *Newgate-Street*.

MDCCLVII.

PREFACE.

About ten Years ago I published a small Volume of Observations of the Air, and epidemic Diseases, from the Year 1727 to the End of 1737; and I have now finished another Volume of like Observations, from 1738 to 1747 inclusive: In the latter, I think, I have been somewhat more careful and exact in the History of the reigning Diseases, and the Method of Cure.—However, as it would have been too great an Interruption to the Series of the Observations, to have entered into particular Disquisitions on the Nature and Cure of the several Diseases, there cursorily mentioned, I have reserved them for the following Essays; in which my Way of thinking and acting as to Fevers in general, and those specified in particular, will more fully appear: And this, I hope, will be of some Service to the younger Practitioners, as these Essays are the Result of a pretty large and long Experience, and the Observations were made with the utmost Care and Diligence.—Whatever be the Event, I flatter myself they will be received as the honest Endeavours of a sincere Well-wisher, not only to his Profession, but to all Mankind.

In the following Essays I have frequently referred to both the Volumes of Observations, and in the latter Volume often referred to these Essays; so that, by these Means, I have endeavoured mutually to illustrate both the one and the others.

Though I have all along strictly kept close to Facts and repeated Experience, (and where I have reasoned from these, I have aimed at the justest Analogy); yet I have supported my Doctrine and Practice very frequently by the Authority of the Ancients, particularly *Hippocrates.*—And this I have the rather done, as well knowing of what great Use they were to me in the Course of my Studies and Practice; and also with a View of recommending their frequent Perusal to young Physicians.—But although my Advice perhaps, in this Matter, may have no great Weight; yet I hope, the concurrent Judgment of the greatest Masters in our Profession will be duly regarded.

I will not take upon me to say, a Person cannot be a good Physician without consulting that great Oracle of Physic, and reading, the Ancients; but this let me say, He will make a much better Physician for so doing: And I believe, few, if any, ever made any considerable Figure in the Profession, who had not studied them.—Indeed *Hippocrates* hath been accounted the very Father of Physic, and the Plan, which he laid down, as the *Basis* of all true and solid Medicine: And it hath been constantly held in the highest Veneration by all his Successors, at least by all those, who were capable Judges of the Matter.—The Reason of which is evidently this, that he studied Nature with the greatest Care and Assiduity, and copied and followed her too with the greatest Exactness; so that his Observations have been found perfectly just through all succeeding Ages.

It is not in Physic only, but in several other Arts, that the Study of the Ancients is of the utmost Advantage, and is universally acknowledged to be so.—Whoever would excel in Poetry, Sculpture, Statuary, *&c.* must always consult the Works of the ancient Masters in these respective Arts, as the most perfect Models, and most just Copiers of Nature; and it is not in Poetry only, but in Physic also, that *Horace's* Advice is good.

——— ——— *Vos exemplaria Græca*
Nocturna versate manu, versate diurna.

In Truth the Ancients were not only Men of vast Genius, but of the greatest Diligence and unwearied Application (the *Roman* Historians have always in the Character of their great Men *incredibilis industria, diligentia singularis*); who kept their Eyes steadily fixed on what they would describe, and gave us the true Picture and naked Truth of Things; which is infinitely more beautiful than all the affected Daubing and Flourishes of a modern luxuriant Imagination: The more just the Description, always the more excellent: What is a Portrait good for, that is not like the Original?—As Nature herself, the more accurately viewed, is the more admired; so he that gives us the truest Copy of her Face, will ever be deemed the greatest Master. In this *Hippocrates* so greatly excelled, that he had the united Applause of the Nations around him, nay they even paid him divine Honours; for by this he was enabled to heal, as well as to know and describe Diseases.—I am fully persuaded, had his Method been strictly followed by succeeding Physicians, the Art of Healing would have long ere this Time been carried to a much greater Height than it is at present: Which hath by no Means kept Pace with the many and great Discoveries, that have been made since (especially within this and the last Century) in Natural Philosophy, Anatomy, the *Materia medica*, and Chemistry.—Indeed as Man is by Nature mortal, it is impossible that Art can make him immortal: but surely it is very possible it may supply something more exact and determinate than we have at present.

From the Days of *Galen*, and indeed long before, vain *Hypothesis*, the Love of Novelty, the Fashion and Faction of Physic too often led its Professors devious, and attached them to Error; and, it is too well known, the same Misfortunes still attend us. However it must be acknowledged, that all the sober, regular, judicious Practice hath been always consonant to the *Hippocratic* Doctrine; as hath been shewn at large by the learned Dr. *Barker* in his late Essay, to which I refer the Reader, and to Dr. *Glass's* ingenious Commentaries for a Scheme of the Practice of *Hippocrates.*

I am so far from blaming a rational Theory in Physic, that I think it the *Basis* of all just and regular Practice; but then it should be, as *Hippocrates* adviseth, *Κατὰ φύσιν θεωρέων**–If ever Physic is to be improved, it must be in such a Manner, and not by *chimerical Hypotheses*, nor rash unwarrantable Quackery.—A diligent Study of the Ancients therefore, and a thorough Acquaintance with the Laws of the animal Œconomy, as rationally delivered by some of the Moderns, should be the Business of every Physician.—But some are more expeditiously popped into the World.—To be the Favourite of a great Man, (or, what is rather better, of a great Woman) to be the Tool or Fool of a Party with a splendid Equipage, and no small share of Assurance; these are Qualifications, which finish the Doctor, to the Reproach of the Profession, and the Danger of the Society.

Celsus hath been justly stiled the *Latin Hippocrates*, not only as having translated an infinite Number of Passages from the divine old Man into his Works, but also as having generally followed his Method and Medicine.—His *Latinity* is most elegant, his Physic and Surgery surprisingly just†.

**De Vict. acut. Sect.* xlvi. *Edit. Lindeni.*

†Although I am far from thinking that Celsus was a Practitioner of Physic, in the common Sense of the Words, as *Asclepiades, Themison,* and *Cassius* were; yet he had certainly well studied it, and diligently perused the most considerable and best Authors then extant in Physic and Surgery—chiefly, perhaps as a Philosopher, who made the whole Study of Nature his Business, like the Sages of old, by whom as *Celsus* himself says,—"*medendi Scientia Sapientiæ Pars habebatur, ut et Morborum Curatio et Rerum Naturæ Contemplatio sub iisdem Auctoribus*

No one hath more closely followed *Hippocrates* than* *Aretæus Cappadox*, so far as to have affected his very Words and Stile:—His

nata fit—ideoque multos ex Sapientiæ Professoribus peritos ejus fuisse accepimus."—And therefore *Columella* very justly stiles him *universæ Naturæ Vir prudens*—for indeed he not only wrote of Medicine, but of Agriculture, the Diseases of Cattle, *&c.*

That he was even conversant in the Practice of Physic and Surgery is pretty evident from his Books *de Medicina*, in which he gives a very judicious Account of Diseases, and the Method of Curing them, and very exact and particular Directions in Chirurgical Operations, even to the minutest Circumstances of Dressing and Bandages; insomuch that it seems very probable, that he actually performed himself, or, at least, had been very often present at such Operations.

Besides, he appears to have been very well acquainted with the *Materia Medica*, and Method of Composition, and hath carefully laid down particular Directions relating thereto, and a precise Account of the Weights, and their Subdivisions, by which he would have the Medicines compounded.

It may be said indeed, that he compiled the chief Part of this Work from the most celebrated Authors that preceded him—unquestionably he did so; but then he hath, in very many Places, interposed his own Advice and Opinion, and that too very often contrary to the Sentiments and Directions of his most favourite Authors, *Hippocrates* and *Asclepiades.*

Upon the whole I cannot but think the attentive Reader will find in *Celsus* a great Number of Passages, which will incline him to believe that that Author was very well versed in the Practice of Physic and Surgery.—Several such the learned Dr. *James Grieve* hath cited in the Preface to his Translation of *Celsus*—and I beg Leave to point out a great many more; but, to avoid being tedious, shall only set down the Number of the Pages in *Almeloveen's* Edition of *Celsus* (with which the *Paduan*, published by *Vulpius*, 1722, exactly tallies) where Passages to this Purpose may be found;—had it been necessary, I could have added many more.

Page 4—19—26—29—30—81—89—90—91—96—111—122—129—140—144—150—152—159—165—176—181—194—197—200—204—227—230—232—242—249—263—271—296—318—332—338—360—364—393—405—406—408—409—416—426—440—441—446—458—475—477—509—512—517—528—530—546.

*It is pretty surprising that none should take Notice of *Aretæus* before *Aëtius Amidenus*, in the fifth Century; (he is indeed named in the *Euporista* attributed to *Dioscorides*, but few think that Piece to be the genuine Work of that Author:) Neither *Galen*, *Cælius Aurelian*, nor *Oribasius* mention him; though so particular in enumerating all the Physicians of Note, antecedent to, or cotemporary with them.—And yet *Aretæus* seems to have been a very considerable Practitioner, and a Man of great Learning and Judgment:—He affects a very singular stile, using many obsolete Words, *Homeric* and *Hippocratic Phrases*, and the *Ionic Dialect*; which, at the Time he wrote in, was almost intirely disused: For, notwithstanding the Conceit of *Vossius*, he undoubtedly did not write till after the Time of *Nero.*—All this one would think should have made him remarkable; especially if he

Descriptions of Diseases are admirable, and his Method of Cure greatly judicious.

Galen should be read by all that would consult the most laboured and exact *Commentator* upon *Hippocrates*: Besides he abounds with an immense Number of fine and useful Observations in all Parts of Physic, and was the first that gave us any particular Account of the Pulses, their Difference and Signification: It is Pity there is so much of the *Peripatetic* and *Periphrastic* in him. The World would probably receive a judicious Abridgment of his Works with no small Satisfaction.

Had *Cælius Aurelianus* written in the Stile of *Celsus*, he would have been an invaluable Author.—As it is, we are vastly indebted to him, for the whole Doctrine of the *Methodists*, particularly of the judicious *Soranus*; as well as for the Sentiments of the Ancients on very many Disorders, which otherwise would have been wholly lost

practised in, or near *Rome*; which is not improbable, as he advises *Roman* Wines to the Sick; particularly the *Falernian, Surrentine, Signine*, and those of *Fundi*.

But further, *Galen* and *Aëtius* quote from *Archigenes* several Passages, which are exactly the same, as to Sense, Doctrine, Method of Cure, and Manner of Expression, with what we find in *Aretæus*; only the latter gives them the *Ionic* Turn.—They both coincide in recommending some particular Medicines, which are scarce to be met with in any others, particularly the external Use of *Cantbarides*; which I think is not to be found in any preceding Author, except *Celsus*.

Did *Archigenes* then borrow from *Aretæus*, or the latter from the former?

It is certain, *Archigenes* practised at *Rome* with a very great Reputation, was a very celebrated Physician and Author, and as such is referred to by *Juvenal, Galen, Cælius, Oribasius, Aëtius*, &c.—He is strictly criticised by *Galen*, sometimes censured, sometimes commended, but never reckoned a mere Compiler.—*Aretæus* on the contrary is mentioned by none but *Aëtius* and *Paulus Ægineta*; nay, which is not a little to be wondered at, he is not so much as found in *Photius*'s *Bibliotheca*.—This is really strange, and not easily accounted for, and would incline one to think that *Aretæus* borrowed from *Archigenes*; or rather transcribed and new-modelled him, giving him the *Hippocratic Diction* and *Ionic Dialect*.—Possibly *Aretæus* might do by *Archigenes* something like what *Cælius Aurelian*, not long after, did by *Soranus*: But, if so, he hath vastly much better *græcised Archigenes*, than *Cælius* hath *latinised* (as he calls it) *Soranus*.—Upon this Supposition we need not wonder at finding the *Roman Wines* recommended in *Aretæus*, though he might practise and write in *Cappadocia*, or any where else, at the greatest Distance from *Rome*—But these are my poor Conjectures.—Be the Matter as it will, in *Aretæus* we have a most valuable Work, a most accurate Description of Diseases, and in general a very proper and judicious Method of Cure; and it is greatly to be lamented, that the Work comes so maimed to us.

to us.—Notwithstanding his *Barbarisms*, his Description of Diseases is most just and admirable.

One of the Ancients more I would particularly recommend, and that is *Alexander of Trallis*, who in most Things indeed follows *Hippocrates* and *Galen*, and generally gives them the Epithet of *θειότατοι*: But yet he hath an infinite Number of useful Remarks of his own, abounds with many excellent Medicines, and writes in a very judicious and regular Manner.

In the following Essays I have not so much aimed at a particular and methodical Dissertation on the Diseases treated of, as to give a few Hints and necessary Observations as to their Nature and Cure; for this would have made the Work voluminous, which I fear is even now not a little tedious.

I have given few or no *Formulæ*, or *Prescriptions*; for, as *Hippocrates* says, he that knows the Disease, knows what is proper to cure it.—When a Physician knows whether Stimulants or Anodynes, Relaxants or Restringents, Attenuants or Incrassants are indicated; he can be at no great loss how to serve himself of proper Drugs, out of the vast *Materia medica*, which we at present abound with.—He should select a few of the most effectual for his Use of each Sort, and stick to them, and not run into the immense *Farrago*, which some are so fond of: By so doing he will soon be acquainted with their real Virtues and Effects, and readily distinguish between the Symptoms of the Disease, and those caused by the Medicines; which is a thing many Times of no small Importance.—I have really seen in private Practice, and some publick Writings, such a jumble of Things thrown together in one Prescription, that it would have puzzled *Apollo* himself to know what it was designed for:—Not but that there are frequently such *Complications* (and *Contra-indications* too sometimes) in Diseases, as makes some Degree of *Combination* and *Contrast* in a Medicine necessary.

But a *Formula*, or *Recipe* as it is called, can be of very little Service.—Twenty or thirty Grains of Rhubarb shall purge some as much, as twice the Quantity of Jalap will others:— One Grain of the *Theban* Extract, or twenty Drops of the Tincture, will doze one as much, as triple the Dose will another.—Besides the Constitution and Manner of living of the Patient must be considered, in Prescription, as well as the Disease: A sober temperate Person, or one that lives chiefly on Milk, Vegetables, and Water, will by no Means bear such warm Medicines, compound Waters and Spirits, as may be quite proper for those, who have dealt largely in Ragouts and Ratafia.—But this is obvious, and so is this Deduction, that we should always begin with small, or very moderate Doses of all Kinds; and that not only the Physic, but the Drink and Diet of the Sick also should be prudently regulated: For surely what we use by Ounces and Pounds cannot but considerably affect us, as well as what we take by Grains and Scruples. *Hippocrates* and the Ancients were very careful in this particular, and very exact in prescribing a *Regimen*: And in this Respect likewise young Physicians would do well to consult them.—As for those, who will neither read nor reason, but practise by Rote, and prescribe at a Venture; I must seriously advise them, at least, to peruse the sixth Commandment.

CONTENTS.

AN

ESSAY

ON

FEVERS,

And their various KINDS.

CHAP. I.

Of the most simple, more complex, and inflammatory Fevers.

THE great *Boerhaave*, in his admirable *Aphorism de cognoscendis & curandis Morbis*, begins with the Diseases of a simple Fibre; and indeed the only Method, to attain to any considerable Knowledge in any Science, is to begin from the very Elements of that Science; for whatsoever is most simple is more easily understood, than that which is more complex: Method and Perspicuity are the natural Consequence of such a Procedure.

Thus, in examining into the Nature of Fevers, it seems most proper to consider the most simple of the Kind first.—Let us suppose then a Person, both as to his *Solids* and *Fluids*, in perfect Health, engaged in violent Exercise, as by Running, or the like: This, if long continued, will greatly encrease the Velocity, Friction, and Heat of the Blood, which, when considerably above natural, are called a *febrile State.*—Here is then the most simple Fever, arising from nothing but the encreased Action of the *Solids* on the *Fluids*, and the Re-action of the latter on the former; which soon subsides on the Cessation of the Motion, or violent Exercise.

Let us next suppose another perfectly healthy Person, exposed to cold moist Air, by which his Perspiration may be considerably suppressed; hence will follow an encreased Quantity of Humors, and an encreased Effort of Nature to throw them off, and remove the Obstructions: Whence a feverish Habit will follow, which however frequently soon wears off by the kindly relaxing Warmth of a Bed, or the like, assisting Nature's Endeavours.

A third, of an equally good Constitution, drinks too largely of Wine, or other spirituous Liquors; which, encreasing the Quantity of Humors, and also the Motion of the Blood by its stimulating Quality, produces a Fever, which in like Manner soon goes off, by Abstinence, *&c.*

In any one of these Cases, only a simple *Ephemera*, or short Fever, is generated.—But if, in the first Case, the Blood was so violently agitated and rarefied, as that, by its great *Impetus*, and Dilatation of the Vessels, some of the red Globules are forced into the *serous Arteries*; an inflammatory Obstruction would be formed: As we see even externally, when the red Globules are forced into the Vessels of the *Tunica conjunctiva* of the Eye, where only *Lymph* or *Serum* should pass. And if withal the Velocity and Heat of the Blood should be so great, as to dissipate much of its thinnest Part; the Remainder would be left gross and thick, and less fit for a free Circulation through the *Minima Vascula*; and the very Serum would be turned into a Kind of Jelly.—For a Heat, not much greater than the Heat in a common Fever, will coagulate the Serum of the Blood; the Consistence of which Jelly will be in Proportion to the Violence and Duration of the Heat.—Here then, I say, by the mere simple accelerated Motion of the Blood, an inflammatory Fever would be produced, of much longer Duration, and more dangerous Consequence.—If the Inflammation seizes the Lungs, a Peripneumony; if the *Pleura*, a Pleurisy; if the Brain, or its Membranes, a Phrenzy is generated.—And these Disorders prove much more severe, where, antecedent to this violent Motion of the Blood, there was a great Strength of the Fibres, and a great Density and Quantity of Blood.

If in the second Case, the Obstruction of the Pores and Perspiration be very considerable, the Fibres strong and tense, the Blood much in Quantity and very thick, Fevers of the same Kind ensue.

If in the third Case, to tense Fibres and much viscid dense Blood, a great Quantity of Wine, or other stimulating Liquors, be added; both the Quantity and Velocity of the Blood may be so greatly encreased, as to bring on a dangerous acute Fever, which too often follows drunken Debauches.

Now as any one of the above Causes may singly produce a Fever; on the Concurrence of two, or all three, a more violent one, *cæteris paribus*, will arise. Thus, from cooling too suddenly after vehement Exercise, as by exposing the Body to very cold Air, and stopping the Sweat and Perspiration at once, a very dangerous inflammatory Fever will come on; which will be much more violent, if the Blood had been heated and encreased by a large Quantity of any spirituous Drink immediately before.—By the bye, nothing so effectually carries off the ill Consequences of a drunken Bout, as keeping warm, and lying long in Bed *to soak it out*, as they call it.

Now by considering the proximate Causes of these Fevers, the Method of Cure is very obvious, which is by lessening the Velocity, Quantity, and Acrimony of the Blood as soon as possible.—But nothing so soon abates the too rapid Motion, Quantity, and Heat of the Blood as Bleeding; for by this Means the red Globules of the Blood and *Vis motrix* are lessened.—By Bleeding *ad Deliquium*, as *Galen*, and some of the ancient Physicians, did in inflammatory Fevers, the Blood's Motion almost quite ceases for a short Time.

Bleeding therefore is certainly the first *Intention* in the Cure of Fevers, that arise from too great a Quantity, and too rapid a Motion of the Blood; and the longer it is neglected, the more viscid and acrimonious is the Blood rendered, by dissipating its more thin Part, condensing the red Globules, and heating the Serum to such a Degree, as to turn it into a Kind of Jelly.—And, by exalting the animal Salts and Oils to a greater and greater Degree of Acrimony (which is always in Proportion to the Intensity and Duration of the Heat) the whole Mass grows putrid at length, and unfit for animal Uses.—Besides, whatever Obstructions may be formed either in the extreme Branches of the *sanguine*, or Beginings of the *serous Arteries*, are apt to be more and more radicated by the too violent Motion of the Blood.—So that the Neglect of Bleeding, at the Begining of any acute Disease, is very often never to be compensated in the subsequent *Stadia* of the Fever; when the *Impaction* of the obstructing Matter is so far advanced, and the Thickness and Viscidity of the Humors so great, as to elude the Force of all Manner of Attenuants and Diluents.

In general, the Quantity of the Blood to be taken away is to be determined by the Strength of the Patient and his Pulse; by the Intenseness of his Fever, Heat, and the Vehemence of his Symptoms, as to Pain, Difficulty of Breathing, *&c.*—Nay the very *Bulk* of the Person is to be considered also; for certainly *cæteris paribus*, a big strong Man can bear to lose more Blood than a small strong Man.—'Tis safer however to take away too little, than too much at a Time, as the Operation may be so soon and so easily repeated, and as often as may be indicated.—If the Pain, Heat, Difficulty of Breathing, *&c.* abate not after Bleeding, it shews the Necessity of drawing more Blood.

And here let me caution the younger Practitioner not to be deceived by an *oppressed Pulse*, which is often the Consequence of too great a Fulness of Blood; this is manifest, by the Vibrations of the Artery becoming more free and strong after Bleeding in such Cases, as daily Experience evinces.—If he is doubtful in the Case, let him apply his Finger to the Pulse in the other Arm, while the Patient is bleeding; and, if he finds it flag considerably, flutter, or intermit, it is Time to desist; if it beats stronger and more open, he may proceed with Safety and Success.—There are indeed some very apt to faint on Bleeding from a natural Laxity of the Fibres, and Want of that due Elasticity, which should contract the Vessels in Proportion to the Evacuation.—These should be bled in a *recumbent Posture*, and the Orifice may be frequently stopped for a short Time, whereby Fainting will be in a great Measure prevented.—These Persons, though they have too lax Fibres and Vessels, are often plethoric, and of Course require Bleeding; especially where the Load of the Humors begins to overbear the Power of the Heart, which is the common Case in an oppressed Pulse.

Bleeding not only lessens the Quantity and Velocity of the Blood, but it also makes Room for the Entrance of diluting Liquors into it.—Proper Dilution is absolutely necessary in all Fevers, especially in the ardent and inflammatory; for in these the Blood is rendered too thick and viscid by the Dissipation of the thinnest Parts of it, and the remaining Serum is more and more incrassated, or jellied, by the great and continued Heat: So that cooling, thin, diluting Liquors are necessary to supply the continual Waste of the Lymph and Serum, and to keep the whole Mass in a due Degree of Fluxility.—These in general, should be of the acescent, and somewhat also of the saponaceous Kind. Of the former, as they are very cooling, and prevent the Encrease of the alcalescent Acrimony of the Humors, which would otherwise be continually advancing by the great Friction and Heat of the Blood:) for the animal Salts are greatly exalted, and made more corrosive, by the feverish Heat, and the animal Oils are by the same cause turned rancid at length, and highly acrid: The sweetest Oils, or Butter, by great Heat, become vastly caustic.—Of the latter, as they not only dissolve the *Lentor* better, but also keep the Humors more properly mixed, by uniting the Salts, Sulphurs, and Waters more intimately with the Blood. I have often known pure Water, drank plentifully in acute Fevers, rendered almost as pale and insipid as when drank; (which, by the Way, is a very dangerous Symptom.) Water, as Water, will not unite with oily Liquors; so that when the Serum of the Blood hath been jellied by Heat, and its oily Part exalted, and encreased, by melting down the Fat in the *Membrana adiposa*, &c. it is no Wonder that plain Water neither mixes well with the Blood, nor proves an effectual Diluent. Hence therefore follows the Necessity of mixing something saponaceous with it, as Sugar, Syrup, Jellies, or *Rob* of Fruits, as Currants, Rasberries, Cherries, or the like.—Juice of Lemons, or Oranges, by mixing a little Sugar with it, and a proper Quantity of Water, becomes a very grateful Drink, and answers the Intention of a Diluent both acid and saponaceous.

Besides the Use of Diluents as to the Humors of the Body, no small Advantage will arise from them as to the Fibres and Vessels, which they tend to relax; especially when they are drank somewhat warm.—Now too great a Tension of the Fibres, *&c.* is naturally concomitant to great Velocity, Heat, and Density of the Blood, which always attend, or rather are the very Essence of an inflammatory Fever.—Every one knows what tepid Bathing will do externally; and it may be easily supposed that subtepid Diluters internally will have an analogous Effect.—In all these Views, the Blood is rendered less rapid, less viscid, and in Consequence, less hot; which are Matters of the highest Import in the Cure of ardent and inflammatory Fevers. It may be added, that obstructed Capillaries, and obstructed Perspiration, are by such Means most safely and effectually remedied, the Humors being rendered *fluxile*, and the *minima Vascula permeable.* For it is to be noted, that where gentle and general Sweats follow plentiful Dilution, with Liquors of a cooling relaxing Nature, they are commonly critical, and soon carry off the Fever. I say, gentle Sweats; for profuse ones should never be encouraged in the Begining of Fevers, as they drain off the thinnest Part of the Blood, and leave the Remainder too thick, viscid, and apt to obstruct.—In a particular Manner I have often observed them of the highest ill Consequence in the Begining of Pleurisies,

Peripneumonies, and the Small-pox.—And for the same Reason, profuse Discharges by Stool, and thin Urine, are hurtful.

But the most pernicious Method of raising Sweats in the Begining of Fevers, is by giving hot volatile alexipharmac Medicines, stoving up the Patients in hot Air, and smothering them almost with Loads of Bed-cloaths; for these encrease the Motion and Heat of the Blood already too violent, and add Fewel to the Fire: Nay, very often, they are so far from raising Sweat, that they prevent it, by hurrying on the Blood with too great Rapidity to give off any natural and regular Secretions.—It is well known, the higher the Fever, the less the Excretions by Sweat, Urine, Saliva, and the like.—

Certainly, if mere encreased Motion of the Blood can bring on a Fever, whatever will encrease that Motion will continue and augment it, which these Methods and Medicines are known to do.

For these Reasons also Blisters, which throw an acrid Salt into the Blood, and greatly stimulate the Fibres, are very improper in the Begining, at least, of all ardent and inflammatory Fevers.—Yet how often do we see, in the common Practice, a Patient bled largely, then blistered, and forthwith put under a Course of hot alexipharmac Bolusses, Cordials, *&c.*? Which is just as rational as to pull out Part of too large a Fire first, and then forthwith endeavour to quench the Remainder, by throwing on Gunpowder, or Spirit of Wine;—or to lay on Whip and Spur to a Horse on the Fret, when we would stop him: which is really the Case in Blistering, where the oscillatory Power of the Vessels is too great, and the Motion of the Fluids too rapid.

After Bleeding, cooling, emollient, laxative Clysters are of very great Use in the Cure of acute Fevers, even at the very Begining, to bring off the indurated Excrements, which frequently are pent up within the Intestines, and to give a Discharge to any bilious acrid Matter, which might otherwise, in Part at least, be resorbed by the *Lacteals*, &c. into the Mass of Blood.—Besides, they are a Kind of a warm, relaxing Fomentation to the Parts in the *Pelvis* and lower Belly, and both derive from the Head and *Præcordia*, and promote a Discharge of Urine also.

A gentle lenient Purge, likewise, is often of the greatest Service, more effectually to cleanse the intestinal Canal of the *putrid Saburra.* But I would always advise to such as act chiefly in the *primæ Viæ* , as *Manna, Cream of Tartar, Sal catharticus Glauberi,*

Rhubarb, *Tamarinds*, and the like:—All *drastic Purgers* are certainly very pernicious, and so are all the hot *aloetic* Tinctures, Pills, *&c.*—Indeed, all profuse Purging is hurtful, as it drains off too much of the lymphatic Part of the Blood, and thickens the remaining.—When Nature seems to have too great a Tendency that Way, first a Dose of *Rhubarb*, then a little of the *Species è Scordio*, with a *diacodiate* Anodyne, or the like, may be proper.

In Deed, little more seems necessary in the Cure of ardent inflammatory Fevers, than proper and well-timed Evacuations, and plentiful cooling Dilution, with a few nitrous Medicines, and the acid saponaceous Juices of Vegetables; for these not only tend to keep the Blood in a due Degree of Fluidity, but also to prevent its running into a putrid State:—In giving these freely, we do but follow Nature (our best Guide) that earnestly demands them.—For how averse soever she may be to Meat in Fevers, she ardently desires Drink; and it is a Symptom of very bad Omen when she doth not, till the Fever considerably abates, at least.

If, from any of the above Causes, an inflammatory Fever should seize a Person that had an antecedent sharp State of Humors, the Fever would prove much the more violent; because the acrimonious Salts would act as so many *Stimuli*, accelerate the Blood's Motion, and produce a speedier and greater Putrescence of it.—Hence therefore the utmost Necessity of Dilution in such Cases, to dissolve and wash off the Salts offending, (for nothing but a watery *Menstruum* will dissolve Salts) and likewise Medicines opposite in Nature to the peccant Acrimony.—But the Diluters also should have something of the Saponaceous in them, for Reasons hinted at above; especially when the oily Parts of the Blood are greatly encreased by the Melting down of the Fat by the Heat of the Fever: which often happens to a surprising Degree, and very suddenly, in some very fat Persons, and which continually grows more and more acrid and rancid, and requires some saponaceous *Medium* to unite it with the aqueous Parts; otherwise it produces the most fatal Obstructions, and highest Degree of Acrimony.

As to the Manner of Dilution, I think the Sick should be allowed to drink as freely, and as often as they please, but not forced to load their Stomachs with two large Draughts at a Time; which create a *Nausea*, Indigestion, and Wind, with great Anxiety and Restlessness, and, in the Event, Vomiting, or Purging.

The Practice of *Asclepiades* was in Nothing more monstrous

than in denying all Manner of Drink to the Sick, for the first three Days of the Fever: And he is very far from keeping up to the Rule he lays down, of curing *tuto, celeriter, & jucundè*; when, as *Celsus* says, *convellebat vires ægri luce, vigilia, siti ingenti, sic ut ne os quidem primis diebus elui sineret. Lib.* iii. *Cap.* 4.—I am sure that he did not learn this from the great *Hippocrates*, nor from Reason, Nature, or Experience.—But this Man from a *Declaimer* turned *Physician*, and set himself up to oppose all the Physicians of his Time; and the Novelty of the Thing bore him out, as it frequently doth the *Quacks* of the present Time; and ever will, whilst the Majority of the World are Fools.

I think smaller Draughts, frequently given, the best Way of Dilution: For, of the same Quantity of Liquor drunk in a certain Time, more is like to be imbibed by the absorbing Vessels, planted thick from the Mouth to the Stomach, by frequently sipping it down, than if swallowed at once in a full Draught; because it is in this Way more frequently, and much longer applied to these Vessels.—Besides, when swallowed, the Action of the Stomach and Intestines is more effectual in squeezing it into the Lacteals and mesaraic Vessels, when in small Quantities, than when they are, as it were, deluged with the Liquor.

Moreover, Dilution and Relaxation may be further carried on by emollient Fomentations, tepid Baths, cooling lenient Clysters, *&c.*—Bathing of the Arms and Hands, Legs and Feet, and also of the *Hypochondria*, is of very great Service in Fevers of the inflammatory Kind; (the good Effects of which I once experienced on myself;) but the *Fotus* should not be much hotter than the present Temper of the Body, which may easily be adjusted by a *Thermometer.* This Method not only supplies the Blood with Moisture through the absorbing Vessels, but also greatly tends to open the osbtructed, and produce a general Relaxation of Fibres, now commonly too rigid. In very dry *strigose* Constitutions, it cannot but be of the greatest Service.—The Skins and Bladders of Animals, when very dry, will transmit nothing; but, when moistened, Water, *&c.* will pass through their Pores.—And the Drinking frequently of tepid, emollient Liquors is at the same Time a Kind of internal relaxing *Fotus* to the *primæ Viæ, Præcordia, &c.* which is of no small Consequence, especially in Inflammations of the Lungs, Pleura, *&c.*—I shall only further add on this Head, that this was the Practice of the Ancients, who gave little else in Fevers, besides thin watery Diluents, *Ptisan* or Barley-water, *Hydromel, Oxymel,* &c. and used very frequent Fomentations and Clysters.

As encreased Velocity of the circulating Humors will of itself bring on a Fever, all Causes that encrease the Blood's Motion will encrease the Fever; the Strength of the Fever therefore will be in a compound *Ratio* of the moving Powers, *viz.* strong tense Fibres, much dense rich Blood, and many acrid Salts in it, which stimulate the Heart and Arteries to more frequent and vehement Contractions.—The large Use of very salt and spiced Meats will raise a feverish Heat, even in the most healthy.

On the contrary, the weaker and more lax the Fibres, the thinner and poorer the Blood, the less vehement the Fever.—This is the Case in what we call *slow*, or *nervous Fevers*; which are generated by low, watery, unwholesome Diet, crude washy Fruit, rainy warm and wet Seasons, long and great Anxiety of Mind, Dejection of Spirits, *&c.*—Here indeed a Kind of *Lentor*, or *Ropiness* of the Humors, is also generated, and is a proximate Cause of the Disease; but it is not of the inflammatory Kind (or what the Ancients called *Phlegma phlegmonodes*, which is particularly inherent in the red globular Parts of the Blood) for it subsists chiefly in the serous and lymphatic Vessels, which hence become obstructed; and from such a poor ropy State of the Blood few animal Spirits are generated, and they are irregularly secreted and distributed: hence the nervous Symptoms, which denominate the Fever.—And yet as there are Obstructions formed, the stagnant Lymph grows more and more acrimonious, which brings on more or less of a Fever, known by the Quickness of the Pulse, irregular Heats, Chills, *&c.*—All the Humors of the Body grow more and more corrosive, the longer they stagnate; even hydropic Swellings of the Legs, though at first as cold as Marble, become at last highly inflamed, the Humors at length so very acrid as to produce an Erysipelas, Vesications, Ulcers, *&c.* as is often observed at the Close of Dropsies.

Now as the Seat of *these Fevers* seems chiefly in the *ultima Vascula*, or the serous and lymphatic Arteries, and perhaps in the very Origin of the Nerves; and as they are always attended with too great a *Flaccidity* and *Torpor* of the Nerves and Fibres, and the Obstructions lie more remote from the great Road of the circulating Blood; it is no Wonder they are not so easily affected by Medicines and so readily removed, as if their Cause lay more particularly in the sanguineous Vessels.—Besides it must be considered, that the

Nerves and Fibres are not presently restored to their due Tone.—Hence we in Fact see that this Kind of Fevers is both longer in forming, and much longer in being carried off, than a common inflammatory Fever.

These two Sorts of Fevers seem to have in a great Measure opposite Causes, and in consequence very different Symptoms and Effects.—Let us consider some intermediate febrile State, which will elucidate this whole Affair. Turn we therefore our Thoughts on an intermittent Fever.

CHAP. II.

Of intermitting Fevers.

THE common procatarctic Causes of Agues are a moist, foggy *Atmosphere* exhaling from a swampy, morass Soil, or a Continuance of cold, rainy, thick Weather; hence in low, fenny Countries Agues are *endemic*, and in such Seasons *epidemic*. By such Constitutions of the Air the Fibres are too much relaxed, and regular Perspiration obstructed, which soon create a *Lentor* of the Blood, and that Obstructions and some Degree of Stagnation in the ultimate Branches of the *sanguineous Arteries*; as is manifest from the Coldness, Paleness, and Lividity of the Fingers, Nails, Lips, *&c.* which immediately precede and begin the *Rigor* of *an aguish Paroxysm.*—The Blood hence recoils upon the Heart, and all the Powers of Nature rouse up to remove the Obstructions; which are soon carried off by the hot Fit, in Sweats, turbid Urine, *&c.*—We see a Kind of aguish Paroxysm brought on by Bathing in very cold Water; Paleness, Coldness, Shivering, a Stoppage of the Blood in the *cutaneous Arteries*, and Repulsion towards the Heart; you are no sooner out of the Bath than the Heart, Arteries, *&c.* overcome the Resistance from the precedent *Constriction*, and bring on an universal *Glow* of Heat. But, if the Person bathed be weak, the Water very cold, and the Continuance in it long; he may die in the cold Bath, as a weakly Patient may in the cold Fit, (which commonly happens, when the Disease proves mortal) the Heart not being able to overcome the Resistance.

If the Fibres are pretty strong, the *Lentor* and Obstructions not very great, the Paroxysm easily wears off by this Effort of Nature.—But if the *Lentor* and Obstructions are great; the Fibres strong and more tense; the Fever runs very high in the hot Fit, and is readily changed by wrong Management into an *acute Continual.*—Indeed it is observable that some epidemic Agues, in some Constitutions, at first put on the Appearance of ardent Fevers, and then break into Quotidians, or Tertians; and it is not uncommon for a Quotidian, or Tertian, to be changed by a very hot Regimen at the Begining, as volatile Spirits, Brandy, Pepper, Snake-root, *&c.* (which are too often quacked upon the poor Patient) into an inflammatory Fever with Phrenzy, Pleurisy, or Peripneumony.—So that the Constitution of the Solids and Fluids, in some Kinds of Agues, seems not greatly different from that of inflammatory Fevers.—I well remember, that the *catarrhal Fever*, which spread through all *Europe* under the Name of *Influenza* in the Spring, 1743, frequently became pleuritic, or peripneumonic; and as frequently, after two or three Days, ran into a Quotidian, or Tertian: the Difference of the Constitutions of the Patients, *&c.* thus altering the Face and Nature of the Disease.

Sometimes quotidian, semi-tertian and tertian Fevers, are very rife and cotemporary with epidemic Pleurisies, and Peripneumonies; as particularly in * 1744:—The cold Season, in some Constitutions, bracing up the Fibres so high, and condensing the Blood into such a Degree of Viscosity, as to bring on these inflammatory Fevers on taking Cold, or other Accidents;—whilst, on Persons of a more lax System of Nerves and Fibres, and more weak, watery Humors, it only raised the Powers of the oscillatory Vessels so high, and warmed the Blood so much, as to carry off the ill Consequences of deficient Perspiration, and ropy heavy Juices, by repeated Fits of a regular Intermittent.—Thus we often see Persons of low Spirits, and a leucophlegmatic Habit of Body, raised into a feverish Disposition by the Use of warm invigorating Medicines, Chalybeates, *&c.* And if this Turn of Nature be well managed, it generally ends in their perfect Recovery.—If you can change a slow nervous Fever into a regular Intermittent, you soon cure your Patient.

But further, I have more than once known Pleurisies, Peripneumonies, and inflammatory Rheumatisms, reign very much in a cold,

* *Vid. Obs. nostr. de Aere & Morb. Epidem. Vol. II. Martio, Aprili, Maio, 1744.*

dry Spring, and a great Number of Intermittents succeed them in the following warmer Months; the Heat abating the Rigidity of the Fibres, and resolving in some Measure the Viscosity and Density of the Blood: Whereas had the Solids continued more tense, and the Blood more dense and viscid, inflammatory Fevers would have been the Consequence, on taking Cold, or the like; which now only produced an aguish Disorder.

Regular *vernal Intermittents* have many Times very salutary Effects, by breaking the *Lentor* and *morbid Cohesions* of the Blood; as a Storm purges a thick foggy Atmosphere. The invigorating Power of the advancing Spring, and the encreasing genial Warmth and Dryness of the Air, by rarefying and attenuating the heavy, sizy Humors, and opening the Pores, are the Reasons why vernal Agues go so easily off at the Approach of Summer. And probably the enlivening, attenuating Influences of the growing Spring, actuating the Powers of Nature to throw off the heavy, ropy *Colluvies*, that in some may be considerably amassed during a cold moist Winter, may be one Reason, at least, of the Frequency of Agues in the Spring Season.—It is certain, all Nature at that Time of the Year undergoes a Kind of *Orgasm*; even the torpid Vegetables regain fresh Life, and their concreted Juices resume new Motion.

It appears from* Experiments, that the Blood in Quotidians is more dense and tenacious than in Tertians, in Tertians than in Quartans; so that in Quotidians, *cæteris paribus*, it comes nearest an inflammatory State: And it is commonly noted, that if the Fever, from a regular Tertian, runs into a Semi-tertian, or Quotidian or greatly anticipates the Time of the regular Paroxysm; a remittent, or continual Fever is forthwith the Consequence.—And this is too often effected by a very hot Regimen, or a too hasty Use of the Bark.—Indeed we very frequently see that Quotidians, and double Tertians, (which, by the bye, are oftentimes the same Thing) will not bear the Bark, at the Begining; till the saline Draughts, proper diluting Attenuants, and, in some Cases, Bleeding, Purging, and Vomiting have been made Use of.—In Truth, I never think it prudent, in such Kinds of Intermittents, to give the Bark, in any Form, till after four or five Paroxysms at least, and after having drawn more or less Blood from Persons pretty much inclined to the plethoric;—and this Method is more especially to be observed in vernal Agues.—I must further note, that as nothing is more effec-

* *See Dr.* Langrish's *Modern Theory, &c. Chap.* V.

tual in curing Agues than well-timed Vomits, and those too repeated; (as Nature shews us, by making this one of her constant Efforts in the Paroxysm) so previous Bleeding makes them much more safe, in full sanguine Habits, especially when given in the Paroxysm; which is frequently practised with great Success.—Nor is this a new Practice; for *Celsus* advises, *cum primum aliquis inhorruit, & ex horrore incaluit, dare ei oportet potui tepidam aquam subsalsam, & vomere eum cogere.* Lib. iii. Cap. 12.

We see then that some Kinds of Agues border too near on the inflammatory State, and require a cool Regimen, proper Dilution, and, many Times, Bleeding to some Degree, as well as other Evacuations. I have known it necessary to join Nitre to the Bark during the whole Process of Cure, and even sometimes to suspend its Use for a Day or two, and give Salt of Wormwood and Juice of Lemons with Infusion of Chamomile-flowers and *Sevil*-orange Rind, or the like.—If an Intermittent runs into an inflammatory continual Fever, Bleeding and a gentle cool Purge will soon reduce it to its *Type*.

But as some Intermittents are apt to run up into an inflammatory Fever, far the greater Number, especially in the autumnal Season, are disposed to sink into low irregular Remittents, putrid or slow nervous Fevers. It is not a very rare Thing to find a Quotidian fall into a Tertian, thence into a Quartan and at last end in a Dropsy; and this particularly in some Seasons and Places. This evidently shews that the Fibres grow more and more enervate, and the Blood very vapid and watery.—Even vernal Tertians, which oftentimes cure themselves in a favourble Season, prove many Times exceeding obstinate in wet, rainy Summers, and the Patients are exceeding apt to relapse on the slightest Occasions: This was particularly observable in the wet, cold Summers of 1734 and 1735*.—In such Cases I have known the daily Use of the Flesh-brush, and frequent cold Bathing, of very great Use in preventing Relapses.—Perhaps it is the Winter-cold, bracing up the Fibres, that commonly puts a Stop to Agues in that Season; for it hath been noted, that they are often very stubborn in a warm moist Winter.

Improper Evacuations by Bleeding and Purging, an unwholsome, gross glutinous Diet, vapid ropy Drinks, as stagnant heavy Water, foul Beer, and the like, render these Agues very *anomalous*, obstinate and dangerous, and make them frequently degenerate

* *Vid. Obs. nostr. de Aere & Morbis Epidemic. Vol. I.*

into malignant, putrid, or slow nervous Fevers; otherwise they end in Dropsies, Jaundice, or universal Obstructions of the *Viscera* of the *Abdomen*, and frequently in Diseases of the *Genus nervosum.*—In a Word whatever takes down the Spring of the Fibres too much, and weakens the *Crasis* of the Blood, will be productive of these Mischiefs; and this especially, when due Perspiration is frequently interrupted by cold damp Air, Want of due Exercise, gross heavy slimy Diet, as Fish, Lettuce, Cucumbers, and other watery insipid Fruits, which are known to suppress the Perspiration greatly.

These Observations then evidently shew the Necessity of using a warm, invigorating attenuating Regimen in the Cure of Agues, which affect Persons of a lax Habit of Body, and a poor thin Blood; in a particular Manner when a wet, foggy Atmosphere prevails.—Under such Circumstances the *Cortex* of *Peru*, however good and carefully chosen, frequently proves ineffectual, unless assisted with proper Alexipharmacs, as *Rad. Serpentar. Virgin.—Contrayerv. Myrrh, Camphire*, &c.—After four or five Paroxysms, warm Chalybeates may be added with very great Success.—But never be too hasty in giving the *Bark*, or Chalybeates, where the Patient hath a *yellow Cast of the Countenance, a tense Abdomen*, and a very costive Habit of Body.—In which Case *mercurial, saponaceous Deobstruents* with *Rhubarb, Aloetics, regenerate* or *soluble Tartar*, should be premised; nay they may in some Cases be very conveniently joined with the *Bark*.

From the whole then of what hath been said on this Head, it appears that a regular Tertian is a *Medium* between an inflammatory and a slow nervous Fever; and that, on the one Hand, the Constitution of the Solids and Fluids may be so highly wrought up as to fire the Blood into a continual Inflammatory; and that, on the other, it may be so far depressed as to bring on the low *Influent*, or *slow nervous Fever.*—And hence the Cause and Cure of such Fevers respectively seem to be obvious.

Now as every Kind of Fever is a Struggle of Nature to relieve herself from something oppressive, we should always favour her Endeavours by the most proper Means that Reason and Experience suggest. But we should be very cautious, at the Begining especially, how we proceed in spurring on, or bridling her Efforts, till we have well considered the Nature, Quantity, and Quality of the Disease, and the Constitution of the Patient. In order to this it will be highly necessary to make a diligent Examination into these two Things; *1st, the State of the Solids,* and *2dly, that of the Fluids.*

CHAP. III.

Of the State of the Solids.

PROBABLY all that we call Firmness of Body, and Strength of Constitution, is originally owing to the *rudimental Stamina* of our Bodies; and on the strong, or weak, Texture of them, in a great Measure, depends our future prosperous, or adverse Health.—There was indeed a determined Constitution and Strength of Fibres designed by Nature, and any Deviation from it may be called a Disease; which may arise from weakly Parents, Errors in Diet, Exercise, and many other Things: And this Deviation I would have heedfully attended to in Practice.

A due Proportion of *Tensity*, consistent with a proper Degree of *Flexibility*, constitutes the happy *Medium* in which perfect Health consists. Too great a Degree of Rigidity tends to waste the nutritious Juices too suddenly, and ends in a *Marasmus*; as too great a Laxity of the Vessels makes them liable to be overloaded, and brings on a *Leucophlegmatia*, or Dropsy. The former over-digests the animal Fluids, the latter doth not sufficiently assimilate what is taken in by Way of Nutriment.

A very strong elastic Set of Vessels act with great Force on the contained Fluids, and produce much Friction, and of Course great Heat, and withal a constant and large Dissipation of the more subtile and aqueous Parts, which render the Blood-globules, in Proportion, more numerous, more dense and compact, and the Humors in general more viscid; as is evident by the State of the Blood always observable in strong laborious People, which is ever of this Kind.—Where this considerably overbears the Standard of Nature, it becomes *constitutional Disease*, and causes a perpetual Fever, as it were, and at long Run ends in *Atrophy* and a compleat *Marasmus*, if some violent inflammatory Disease doth not snap them off much sooner; and to which they are exceedingly liable, and from which, on Account of the dense viscous State of the Blood, the

Rigidity and Contraction, or *Stricture* of the Vessels, they escape with much greater Difficulty than others of softer Fibres, and a more weak, but fluxile, Blood. There is no Advantage without an Allay; the Rose hath its Prickles; these Disadvantages flow even from the highest Health and Vigor: *Human Frailty!*

In such Constitutions the Use of emollient farinaceous Drinks and Diet is highly proper, and frequent subtepid Bathing, especially in very dry, and very cold Weather.—Where Persons of such a Frame fall into inflammatory Fevers, as Pleurisies, Peripneumonies, or the like, I would always advise great Plenty of tepid, watery, emollient Diluents to be perpetually sipped; by which Means the warm Vapor relaxes the Parts and Passages of the Lungs, and promotes a freer Flow to the Blood through them, and a more easy and copious Expectoration; at the same Time that the Blood is thus most effectually diluted.—Withal Fomentations, emollient and diluting, moderately warm (not too hot) should be applied to the Feet, Legs, Hands, Arms, *Hypochondria* and Breasts; which have oftentimes a surprising good Effect, and are of infinitely greater Advantage and Efficacy than some of the *indigestible Trash of the Shops*, upon which so much *Stress* was formerly laid.

I have known the preposterous Use of the *cold Bath*, on a *Strigose* and a *too rigid Habit* of Body, of exceeding great Detriment; for that even yet augments the *Corrugation* and *Tensity*.—You may generally observe that most, who use the cold Bath, grow somewhat thinner, though more vigorous and active.—Some Years since I was consulted by a Gentleman of a thin scraggy Habit of Body, but of much natural Vivacity of Spirit, and one that constantly used much Exercise, and had long accustomed himself to cold Bathing in the Sea very frequently, even sometimes in very cold Weather: He wasted daily in his Flesh, and at length became weak and very low-spirited.—I judged, that by this Method the fibrous System was overbraced, and that too much of the finer *Lymph*, and even of the *Liquidum nervosum*, was forced off by the Pores, *&c.* For he all this while used a sufficient Quantity of Food, and had no extraordinary sensible Evacuation.—I put him on a soft, relaxing, nourishing Diet, forbad him the Use of the Cold-Bath, and at last sent him to use the Waters at the *Bath*:—The Event was, that he soon recovered much better Health, Spirits and Flesh. Nothing on the contrary more effectually strengthens weak, lax Fibres than cold Bathing: By this weak, flabby, rickety Children are soon invigorated, as it were to a Miracle.—Indeed in the Times of Popery and Ignorance, when the Priests were Knaves, and the People Fools, many a *Well* was sanctified for nothing but pure *cold Water*, the Virtues of which the *Miracle-mongers* wholly attributed to a *Saint* of their own making.

The Doctrine of the ancient *Methodists*, with Respect to the *Strictum* and *Laxum*, if rationally pursued, might be of great Service in the Practice of Physic; though they indeed frequently confounded them both in Theory and Practice. But *Boerhaave* hath made many rational and valuable Observations on the Diseases of too tense, and too lax Fibres, which are of exceeding great Use in Practice.—There seems to be another *Species of Fibres* not taken Notice of, which may be called the *tender*, or *delicate Constitution of the Solids*, which is most readily and highly affected with Pleasure, or Pain; But in which the *Stamina* are so slender, that a very slight Accident breaks them. This is often observed in thin, fair Persons, of a very delicate Frame, but exceedingly lively; in whom the *Spirit* is willing, through the *Flesh* is weak: Such very often fall into an *Hæmoptoe*, or other *Hæmorrhages*, Colliquations, and a pulmonary *Phthisis*, and thence become what is peculiarly called Consumptive.

We have taken a short View of the ill Effects of a too great *Stricture*, or *Tension* of the Solids; let us next cursorily see what Disadvantages arise from their too great Laxity.

Weak Vessels do not sufficiently act on the contained Fluids, they do not sufficiently *comminute, round off*, and *assimilate* the chylous Particles:—Indeed the Chyle itself, where the Organs of Digestion are weak, is never well prepared.—Where the Vessels have a due Tone, and act with Vigor on the nutritious Juices which they receive from the Stomach, *&c.* no chylous irregularly formed Particles are to be found in the Blood after a few Hours from the Repast; but, in weakly *leucophlegmatic* People, they are never, or not till after a very long Time, reduced into Blood-globules, and a proper *Serum.*—Besides in these lax Habits the Blood itself is not sufficiently actuated, and driven on with Force enough to keep a due vital Warmth, nor to work up the Salts and Sulphurs, or Oils, to such a just Degree of *Tenuity*, as may fit them to serve the Purposes of animal Nature; nor are the red Globules of the Blood (the great Principle of Life and Heat) duly compacted, and moulded into a sufficient Roundness and Firmness.—Hence irregular Concretions in the Vessels, a *Lentor*, or *Ropiness* in the *Serum* and *Lymph*, few animal Spirits, and all the Secretions weak and imperfect.—From the whole follow *Cachexy*, *leucophlegmatic* and dropsical Disorders, irregular intermittent and remittent Fevers, or those of the slow nervous Kind; the Humors running into a Kind of Putrescence for Want of due Motion and a Circulation, and stagnating in the *ultima Vascula*, on Account of the Obstructions continually forming from the Want of a due Action of the Vessels, which do not sufficiently agitate, comminute and protrude their Contents.

Now all Humors of the Body, that stagnate, soon begin to corrupt and grow acrimonious, and that too many Times to such a Degree as to bring on Fevers of the worst Kind: For though the Circulation may be very languid, from the Weakness of the contracting propelling Vessels, yet it is sufficient to cause some Degree of feverish Heat from the stimulating Acrimony, and at last a general Putrefaction; witness the *chlorotic Fevers*, which very often prove of exceeding dangerous Consequençe.—Cold hydropic Tumors of the Legs frequently end in a Kind of Erysipelas and Gangrene.

A due Consideration therefore of the State of the Solids is a Matter of high Importance to Physicians, not only in chronic, but also in acute Diseases; for they are generally the primary efficient Causes of the particular States of the Fluids. For Instance, we may naturally conclude that a Man of a robust Constitution, strong, rigid Fibres, and used to much Exercise, hath a dense rich Blood, inclining to such a Degree of Viscidity, as will bring on Inflammations on the Accession of a feverish Disorder; and, of Course, that timely Bleeding is the proper Way to prevent it: On the contrary, that a weak, lax, flabby Constitution hath a poor, thin, watery Blood, and cannot bear Bleeding well, nor large Evacuations.

A diligent Enquiry of this Nature is of vast Concern in the Begining of acute Diseases, particularly in the Small-pox, and other eruptive Fevers; so as to determine one to bleed, or not to bleed.

For Instance, where a strong Man, with a strong Pulse, is seized with violent Symptoms of the Small-pox, it would be unpardonable not to bleed before the Eruption; for we cannot but suppose the inflammatory Fever must run high in such a Constitution; but it would be great Rashness to bleed Persons of a weak, lax Habit, unless some very urgent Symptom demanded it.—Yet how little is this regarded in the vulgar Practice? For some bleed, and vomit, of

Course, upon the least Appearance of an Attack of the Small-pox; whereas others are so fearful of weakening their Patients, that they suffer them to die of the Inflammation, even abstracted from the Virulence of the Disease.

If a Physician hath a previous Knowledge of the Patient, he can be at no great Loss in judging of his Constitution; and therefore *Celsus* rightly pronounces, *cum par scientia sit, utiliorem tamen medicum esse amicum, quam extraneum**. When that is not the Case, hard firm Flesh, dry Skin, great Heat, Thirst, and Colour, hot Breath and violent Pains; with a strong, tense, quick Pulse, are pretty evident Symptoms of strong, very elastic Fibres, and of an ardent or inflammatory Fever.—A weak, quick, soft Pulse, no great Heat, or Colour, little Thirst, pale Urine, a soft Flesh and Skin, clammy, partial, irregular, cold, or profuse Sweats, with Heaviness and Anxiety, rather than severe Pains, and a moist, though perhaps a white coated, or foul Tongue, denote the contrary.—But in Truth these Things are rather to be learned from Experience, than taught by Precept:—Therefore I shall say no more on this Head.

C H A P. IV.

Of the State of the Fluids.

THE State of the Fluids should next be considered, which, in a great Measure, depends, as was said before, on the Condition of the Solids.

There is then, *1st*, a State of the Blood, in which the Humors are too dense and viscous, in which the Blood-globules are in too great Quantity, and too closely compacted or condensed, in which the serous Globules are so likewise.—In a Word, in which the whole Mass of the Fluids is too glutinous, and too apt to concrete into a solid Form.—Persons of vigorous Constitutions, of strong Fibres, that use much Exercise, and a full Diet, are peculiarly subject to this State.—Now when the Blood-globules are very dense, and in great Quantity, and the Vessels very strong and elastic, a great *Momentum of Motion* must be produced in the circulating Fluids, and of

* *Præfat. sub finem.*

Course great Friction, and much Heat, which both dissipates the more fluid Parts of the Blood, and encreases its Viscosity; so that the Residue becomes very glutinous, and less fit to pass the extreme Branches of the capillary Arteries; and hence Obstructions, hence Inflammations.

Besides, great Heat tends to coagulate the *Serum*; a Heat, not much above the common Heat in an ardent Fever, will turn the *Serum* of the Blood into a Jelly, as is found by Experience:—Hence, when blood is drawn off in high inflammatory Fevers, it appears covered over with a thick glutinous Coat, or *Buff*, as it is called; I have seen it in some severe pleuritic and rheumatic Disorders near an Inch thick.—That it is thus formed by the febrile Heat, is manifest; for at the first Bleeding, at the very Begining of the Fever, it shall often appear pretty florid, tho' very dense; whereas on the second, third, or fourth Bleeding, when the Heat hath had a longer Continuance, and been encreased to a greater Degree, it becomes exceeding sizy, and covered over with a very thick Buff:—And indeed, in general, the stronger the Fever, and the Person from whom it is drawn, so much the more thick and tenacious.—And this in a particular Manner happens in Fevers attended with violent Pain, as Pleurisies, Rheumatisms, *&c.*—For the Pain being a *Stimulus*, which greatly encreases the Motion, Friction, and Heat, it *incrassates the Serum* in Proportion to its Vehemence.—And the inflammatory *Size* also sticking in the extreamly small Vessels of the Membranes, *&c.* over-distends them, and produces further Inflammations and Pains; so that they mutually encrease one the other. Tho' this dense State of Blood, in Health, is attended with great bodily Strength, a strong firm Pulse, and much natural Heat; yet, on the Access of a Fever, it produces very violent Symptoms, quickly fatal, unless prevented by timely Bleeding cooling, diluting, emollient Drinks and Medicines.

But further, an Over-fulness of even good Blood is a Degree of Disease, and therefore *Hippocrates** pronounces the *athletic* 'Ε*υεξία* dangerous, and *Celsus* elegantly says from him, that Persons of such a Habit *suspecta habere bona sua debent*†.—Such a *Plethora* not only over-distends the sanguineous Arteries, but also too much dilates the Orifices of the serous and lymphatic Arteries; by which, on the slightest Occasions, the Blood-globules are forced

* *Aphorism* 3. *Sect.* i.

† *Lib. II. Cap.* 2.

into them, and form Obstructions *errore loci,* as it is called: Whence Inflammations and Ruptures of the Vessels frequently follow, particularly in the Brain and Lungs.—Here nothing will relieve equal to Blood-letting, which (if not too immoderate) is so far from weakening, that it Strengthens the Patient, by restoring a due *Æquilibrium* between the Solids and Fluids: The keeping up of which however is a Matter of great Nicety in some Cases and Constitutions; tho', in general, in general, it admits of a considerble *Latitude,* even consistent with Health. Some delicate, florid, plethoric People suffer immediately from a very small Degree of over, or under, Living; and I have known some Men of this Constitution, that have had as regular a *menstrual Discharge,* by some Kind of Hæmorrhage, as the more delicate Sex.—The best bred, and most accurately fed, *Cock,* will not hold his *athletic State* above twenty-four Hours*, and dwindles from it surprisingly soon—*Quia non ultra progredi potest, retro, quasi ruinâ quâdam, revolvitur,* as *Celsus*† says of a plethoric Man.

There is, *2dly,* a Constitution, or Crasis of the Blood, quite opposite to the former, in which there are too few Blood-globules, and those too loosely compacted; and in which the *Serum* is too watery and vapid, and sometimes of a ropy slimy Nature. From this weak pituitous Blood all the Secretions are imperfect, and not sufficiently participant of an animal Nature; the *Bile inert,* the animal Spirits flat and deficient, the *Saliva* a mere *insipid Mucus,* and so on.—Hence universal Indigestion, Weakness, Coldness, Paleness, *Cacochymy,* Dropsy, *&c.*—In a Word, such a slow Motion of the Humors, that at length, for Want of a due Circulation, they run into morbid concretions obstructing the Vessels in some Places, and stagnating in others, where they fall into spontaneous Corruption, productive at last of such a Degree of Acrimony, as to end frequently in Fevers of a very malign Nature, and dangerous Consequence: And this the more so, as the Vessels, in such a miserable Constitution, have greatly lost their Elasticity, and the Blood its most vital Principles:—So that, in the Event, either the *slimy Lentor* stagnates up to the Heart, or the corrupted Humors corrode and destroy the most delicate and essential Parts of the animal Fabric, particularly the *Compages* of the Brain, where

* *See Dr.* Bryan Robinson *on the Food and Discharges of human Bodies, p.* 119.

† *Lib. II. Cap.* 2.

the Humors naturally move exceeding slow, and the Vessels are of the most tender Structure.—Thus as too rapid a Circulation often bursts the minute Vessels; so the Humors, moving too slowly, stagnate, corrupt, and at length corrode them.

These two different States of the Fluids may not improperly be called constitutional, as they naturally follow the respective State of the solids; so as that a strong rich Blood always attends a strong elastic Set of Vessels, and a weak watery Blood a relaxed Habit of Body: where either considerably deviates from the Standard of Nature, it becomes a real Disorder, and is to be duly regarded in whatever concurring Disease happens*.

CHAP. V.

Of the dissolved and putrid State of the Blood.

BUT, besides these, there is moreover a *third State of Blood,* of more dangerous Consequence than either; I mean a State of it, that more immediately tends to *Dissolution* and *Putrefaction*:—This is evidently the Case in some *Scorbutics,* (as they are called) where, without any considerable, antecedent, sensible disorder (more than perhaps a Kind of Lassitude and Languor) Persons have, on a sudden, an Eruption of violet-coloured, livid, or even black and blue Spots all over their Body, and forthwith fall into profuse, and sometimes dangerous and even fatal *Hæmorrhages,* when they have scarce thought themselves, or been thought by others, to be under any Manner of Disorder.—Abundance of Instances of this Kind happen: I have seen a great many both in Children and grown Persons, and frequently foretold the ensuing Hæmorrhage.

Where *Women* have such Eruptions, or black or blue *Vibices,* or large irregular Spots like Bruises, they are always subject to a Vast Overflow of the *Catamenia,* if not to other profuse Hæmorrhages.

* *Ardent and inflammatory Fevers are naturally the Effect of over-elastic and rigid Fibres, and a very dense viscid Blood; as the low and slow nervous Kind are of a too lax State of Vessels, and a weak and thin Blood.—But there are several Diseases, especially those arising from Contagion, which are common to both.*

—Nay when Persons of either Sex are affected with these Appearances, they are apt to bleed excessively from the slightest Wound, and very often without any, from the Gums, Nose, Guts, or urinary Passages.

The Blood of such Persons, when it hath been drawn off, in order to prevent the further Progress of the Hæmorrhage, as was imagined, (which by the Way is very improper, unless there are very manifest Signs of a *Plethora*) always appears a *mere Gore* as it were, not separating into *Crassamentum* and *Serum*, as usual, but remaining in an uniform half-coagulated Mass, generally of a livid, or darker Colour than usual, tho' sometimes it continues long very florid; but it always putrifies very soon. —It is even observable, that the *Breath* of such People most commonly stinks much before the Eruption, and their *Urine* frequently smells very rank; evident Signs of the begining *Putridity* of the Humors; which, growing more and more acrimonious, at length erode the Vessels. For these Kinds of Hæmorrhages often happen to Persons, that have not the least Sign of a *Plethora*, no full, no very quick Pulse, little or nothing of a feverish Habit, not under the Use of violent Exercise; so that they happen from the *Corrosion*, not the *Rupture*, of the Vessels broke open by too great a Quantity and Velocity of the Blood.—In some very tender and delicate Constitutions indeed, a very small Effort will sometimes burst their fine thin Vessels, as is observable in some, who are subject to an *Hæmoptoe*, or Bleeding at the Nose from every small Accident; but these Hæmorrhages are seldom attended, or preceded, with livid, or violet-coloured Eruptions, *&c.*—In these Cases Drawing of small Quantities of Blood is proper, to abate the too great *Impetus* on the tender Vessels, even tho' there may be no apparent *Plethora*.

Tho', I am persuaded, the above-mentioned Hæmorrhages most commonly arise from an *acrimonious State of the Humors*, which breaks the *Crasis of the Blood*, and corrodes the Extremities of the capillary Arteries; yet they sometimes also happen from a too loose Contexture of the Blood-globules, not sufficiently compacted by the Action of the Heart, Arteries *&c.* for Want of which they become *oblate Spheroids*, or irregularly formed *Moleculæ*, instead of *regular Spheres*, and of Course of a greater Diameter, and a less firm *Compages* than natural.—But it appears from microscopical Observations (especially those made with the *Solar Microscope*) that the Bloodglobules, in passing thro' the minutest Ramifications of the sanguineous Arteries, change their globular, into a very oblong Figure frequently, in order to pass thro' these exceeding small Vessels.—And it is easy to conceive how these loosely cohering Globules may be broken in their Passage, as the enlarged Bulk makes their *Transit* more difficult.—Now as these broken Parts are of much lesser Diameter than the original Globules, they may readily enter, and even pass thro' some of the excretory Ducts and transude *per Diapedesin,* as the Ancients called it.—That this is so in Fact seems to appear from the bloody Urine, Stools, and other Hæmorrhages, which sometimes happen without any Manner of Pain, Violence of Motion, or the least Suspicion of the Rupture of any Vessels:—Nay, I have more than once or twice seen in malignant Fevers, and that too where the Motion of the Blood was far from being very rapid, a Kind of * bloody Sweat from the *Axillæ,* tinging the Linnen almost of a *Burgundy* Wine Colour.—And it is observable, that when this Sort of Hæmorrhages happens from the Nose, the matter is a thin *bloody Ichor,* not concreting, as Blood commonly doth from the Nose of Persons in Health, or in an inflammatory Fever, which is generally very thick, shining and florid: Some *chlorotic Girls* are vastly apt to bleed from the Nose, and yet their Blood doth but just colour a linnen Cloth.—The *Petechiæ, Vibices,* or livid *Stigmata,* that very often attend these Hæmorrhages, shew that the Blood-globules are dissolved, or broken down, and enter into the serous Arteries, *Vasa exhalantia, &c.* where sticking fast they form these Appearances.—And I have particularly noted, in some putrid, malignant Fevers, a Kind of yellow, or rather dun *Petechiæ*†, vastly numerous, and of not less fatal Omen than the others: Here the Blood-globules were broken into such small Particles, as to have quite lost their original Colour when combined. Perhaps the fuliginous Sweats, and dark coloured, or black Urine with a livid Sediment, which sometimes happen in Fevers of the malignant Kind, arise from a broken corrupted State of the Blood-globules: I have seen several Times the Urine rendered almost quite black, depositing an immense Quantity of Matter nearly of the Colour of *Coffee-grounds.*—And we are sometimes surprized to see the Face and Hands of the Sick grow *dirty,* and *sooty* as it were, tho' all imaginable Care was taken to keep them clean.

Besides there are some Things that seem to destroy the *Copula*

* *Dr.* Hodges, *of the Plague, observed purple Sweats in it, and some like Blood.*

† *Vid. Obs. nostr. de Aere & Morb. Epidem. Vol. I. Ann.* 1735, *Mart. & Aprili; & Vol. II. Anno* 1740, *Junio.*

of the Blood-globules, and greatly promote the *Secession* of the *six serous Globules,* that compose them, one from another; particularly *Laurel-water,* which makes the *Crassamentum* vastly less dense, and exceedingly more soft and tender than natural, and turns the Serum red, or of the Colour of *Burgundy* Wine, as appears from the curious Experiments* of Dr. *Nicholls* and Dr. *Langrish* †.—the Bite of the Serpent *Hæmorrhous* || causes such a Dissolution of the Blood, that it breaks forth from all Parts of the Body, even the very *Pores,* and kills by an *universal Hæmorrhage.* Possibly *profuse sweats, Diarrhœa, Diabetes,* and Spontaneous Salivations, may arise from a Kind of Dissolution of the serous Globules.—A long and large Use of *Mercury* will turn the whole Mass of Blood into a mere watery *Colluvies.*

But, as I said before, this broken, corrupted State of the Blood-globules is, in general, the Effect of Acrimony. §*Sal volatile oleosum* mixed with Blood fresh drawn, destroys, or dissolves the Globules in less than a Minute;** Spirits of Harts-Horn, taken in large Quantities, will produce Hæmorrhages; and so will frequent and large Doses of Aloetics, as I have again and again observed.—Indeed, such a State of Blood is commonly brought on by acrimonious Diet, Medicines, *&c.*—Thus the salt and half rotten Provisions of Sailors, in long Voyages, cause such a Sharpness and Corruption of the Humors, that they are rendered almost unfit for the common Uses of Life, producing great Weakness, Languors, wandering Pains and Aches, stinking Breath, corroded spongy Gums, black, blue, and sallow Spots, sordid, dark, livid, fungous Ulcers, Gangrenes, *&c.* and such *Scorbutics* frequently fall into petechial Fevers, bloody Dysenteries, Hæmorrhages, *&c.* What is mentioned by the Rev. Mr. *Walter,* in Lord *Anson's* Voyage, is very surprising, *viz.* that the Blood burst forth from the Wounds of some of the *Scorbutics,* after they had been *cicatrised* for twenty or thirty Years.—I have known many a Ship's Company set out on a Cruize in high Health, and yet in two or three Months return vastly sickly, and eaten out with the Scurvy, a third Part of them being half rotten, and utterly unfit for Service.—About four or five Weeks

* *Dr.* Mead *of Poisons, 3d Edit. p.* 270.

† *See his Experiments on Brutes.*

|| *See* Lucan, Dioscorid. Nicander *in* Theriacis, *&c. Dr.* Mead *of Poisons.*

§ *See* Leeuwenhoek. Epist. ad Christoph. Wren. Arcan. Natur.

** Arbuthnot *of Diet, p.* 106.

after they have been out, they begin to drop down one after another, and at length by Dozens, till at last scarce half the *Complement* can stand to their Duty: Particularly I remember, some few Years since, from a Squadron under Admiral *Martin,* we had near 1200 Men put on Shore sick at one Time, tho' they went out very healthy, and returned in about twelve or thirteen Weeks*.

Those who accustom themselves to take largely of volatile and fixed alcalious Salts, Species, and Aloetics, are always subject to these Maladies.—Not a few of those, who took the *alcalious saponaceous Hotch-potch of Mrs.* Stephens, and the *Soap Lees,* for a long Time together, fell into hectical Heats, a hot Scurvy, Hæmorrhages, Dysentery, *&c.*—A remarkable Instance of this lately happened to a Gentleman of the *West of Cornwall,* who for several Years had laboured under a Stone in his Bladder:—He was originally of a tender Constitution, and had taken the *Lixivium,* &c. for several Weeks, till at length his Gums began to grow exceeding spongy, inflamed and livid, at last extreamly sore and putrid, insomuch that the Flesh might be pulled off with the greatest Ease; they bled considerably on the least Pressure, and a thin bloody *Ichor* continually leaked off from them.—Livid Spots also appeared on him, and his legs, and Thighs especially, became vastly sore, and of a Claret Colour, or rather more livid, so that a Mortification was feared. Upon this I was consulted for him by Mr. *Hingston,* a very skilful *Apothecary of Penryn,* who stated his Case.—Apprehending an *alcalescent*; putrid State of the Humors, and a Dissolution of the Blood from the Course he had gone through, and the Symptoms he now laboured under, I advised the Decoction and Extract of the *Bark* with *Elixir Vitrioli,* and subacid Drinks and Diet; which soon took off the Inflammation, Sponginess, and Bleeding of his Gums, and prevented the further Advance of the livid Colour of his Thighs, *&c.* which in a few Days disappeared.—About some two or three Weeks after, a copious Eruption of red, fiery Pustules broke out upon him, which seemed to promise some Advantage.—However, being reduced exceeding weak by a Complication of Disorders, and a cofirmed Hectic, he died quite tabid about a Fortnight or three

* *Upon this I drew up a Proposal for preventing the Scurvy among the Sailors, which I communicated to several Captains and Surgeons of the Men of War. This I afterwards published in the* General Evening Post *in* Octob. 1747, *which was republished in the* Gentleman's Magazine, *&c. for Octob. 1747.—As it hath since been tried with Success, both in the Men of War and Privateers; and, as I am fully convinced of its Usefulness, I again recommend it.* See *Page* 137.

Weeks after.—A very *large Stone was taken out of bis Bladder* after his Death, of the Shape of a Pear, weighing ℥viii ʒss Avoird. the smaller End lay towards the Neck of the Bladder.

It unquestionably appears from Experiments made on the Urine of those that have taken pretty largely of the *Lixivium*, or Mrs. *Stephens*'s Medicines, that the Urine becomes alcalious*, and of Course the Serum of the Blood likewise, from whence it was secreted.—This is indeed a very strong Argument in Favour of the *lithontriptic*, or *dissolvent* Power of the Medicines; as they have undoubtedly this Effect on human *Calculi*, when macerated in them, out of the Body.—But I think, at the same Time, it gives us just Reason to suspect very dangerous Consequences from a long Use of such Things; especially in some tender Constitutions.

It is well known, that volatile-alcali Salts mixed with the Blood, when just drawn, or rather as it runs from the Vein, keep it from coagulating, and hinder it from separating into Crassamentum and Serum, as usual: The Experiment is easy, and every one will find it true on Trial. This very adequately resembles the Blood drawn from the bleeding Scorbutics, and also from most Persons that labour under putrid petechial Fevers, when the Blood is drawn very early in the Disease.

All Humors of the Body, actually putrefied, become a strong Alcali, and putrid Blood loses its Consistence, and soon after its Colour, running into a yellowish dark-coloured *Sanies*—The Blood drawn in some greatly putrid, petechial Fevers hath had this Appearance, and been observed actually to stink as soon as drawn†, as well as the Urine as soon as made; so far was the Putrefaction advanced whilst even Life was still subsisting. The surprisingly great, and speedy Corruption of Bodies, dying of pestilential Fevers with Spots, shews this likewise: I have known such a *Corpse air* ‖ as much, as they call it, in seven or eight Hours, as dead Bodies commonly do in seven or eight Days, and to leak out a most putrid *Sanies* from all the Outlets of the Body:—Which, by the bye, is a Reason why Persons, dying of such Fevers, should be buried very soon.

* *See the Experiments of Dr.* Hartley—Rutty. *Mons.* Morand, *&c. on this Matter.*

† *Vid. Vander Mye de Morbis Bredanis— Morton, Pyretolog. Prolegomen, p.* 26.

‖ *De Aere & Morb. Epidem. Vol. I. Martio,* 1735.

Some Kinds of Poisons, as particularly the *Bite* of a *Viper*, and some other venomous Animals, bring on a very sudden Corruption and Dissolution of the Blood, and turn it into a yellowish *Sanies: Pestilential Effluvia* also soon destroy the *Crasis* of the Blood, and produce an universal gangrenous Disposition in the Humors.—This is evident from the frequent and fatal Hæmorrhages, excessively foetid Sweats, Vomitings and Stools, and the general *Necrosis* that follows, which have been observed in the Plague, and pestilential Fevers, by the best Authors* .—The Hæmorrhages in particular are often vastly profuse and obstinate in the Plague; and I have many Times noted the same in pestilential and petechial Fevers; and the Blood, thus issuing, doth not coagulate† as usual:—All Arguments of the highest Acrimony and Dissolution of the Blood.

The Contagion of the Small-pox seems to affect some Constitutions much in the same Manner, producing Spots, Putrefaction, and Vast Effusions of Blood from several Parts of the body, sometimes even at one and the same Time.—I have seen many Instances in this Disease, where, within four or five Days from the Seizure, Purples have appeared all over the Body, and Hæmorrhages from several Parts in a profuse Manner; particularly the *Uterus*, urinary Passages, and Nose; and the Pustules have turned quite black, a *bloody Ichor* issuing from them in Abundance; and this too where no violent Symptoms of any Kind had preceded.—Little Miss *R—n*, about five Years old, had such a Kind about fourteen Years ago; they came out with scarce any considerable Fever, Pain, Sickness, or the like, yet Spots appeared at the same Time very large, livid and black.—The Pox were but few, some of which about the Lips, internal Parts of the Cheeks, and Tongue, turned very black, and bled pretty largely.—The Child was often taken with a slight *Deliquium*, and forthwith would return to her Play-things as before.—At length she brought off pretty much florid Blood, and some black and coagulated, by Stools, and sunk away insensibly as it were into the Arms of Death, about the ninth Day from the Attack of the Disease.

I lately saw a dreadful Case of this Kind in Miss *B—y*, a young Gentlewoman, who had much fatigued herself in very hot Weather, immediately before the Seizure with the Small-pox, by walking,

**Particularly* Diemerbroek, Hodges, *and the Authors in* Traité de la Peste fait par Ordre du Roy, *Paris* 1744. 4*to*.

† *Traité de la Peste, Part I. p.* 343.

riding, dancing, *&c.*—She had Millions of *truly small* Pox, and a vast Number of black and blue Spots, that broke out all over her Body the third Day inclusive from the Seizure, and her Legs and Thighs appeared quite purple; she bled at the Gums and Nose very largely, and yet at the same Time had a very profuse Discharge of the *Catamenia* about six Days before the regular Period.—She died the sixth Day from the Attack:—She had from first to last an inexpressible Load at her Breast, with vast Anxiety, frequent Faintings, and a vastly quick, fluttering, small Pulse.

It is always a fatal Prognostic, when Spots and Hæmorrhages appear at the very Eruption of the Small-pox, and the Sick seldom, or never, survive the ninth Day of the Disease; the Blood running into immediate Dissolution and Putrefaction. I am persuaded, scarce one in a Thousand recovers under these dreadful Circumstances; especially if the Spots are very livid, black and numerous.—If any Thing is to be done in these deplorable Cases, it must be by timely and duly administering *Acids*, the *Bark* and *Astringent Alexipharmacs*; which certainly have often times exceeding good Effects in petechial Fevers attended with Hæmorrhage.—Dr. *Mead*, in his late elegant Treatise *De Variolis & Morbillis**, hath given us Reason to hope for Success by the Use of these Medicines in the bleeding and petechial Small-pox and also the Method of exhibiting them.

This dissolved State of Blood also often happens in putrid malignant Fevers, arising frequently from *Contagion*; but is sometimes the mere Effect of a Fever seizing Persons of an *acrimonious* State of the Blood and Humors, which is the Case of the *highly scorbutic*: The former acting in an analogous Manner to the Poison of the Viper on the Blood; the latter by the Power of the *saline Spicula* on the Blood-globules, which is now greatly increased by the febrile Motion and Effervescence of the Blood. Thus an inflammatory Tumor in Persons of a good, sweet, sound Constitution suppurates into a *kindly laudable Matter*; in a very sharp State of Humors it turns either into a *gangrenous Sanies,* or *cancerous Ichor.* What the Action of animal Heat and Motion will do, on the Salts of the animal Humors, may be seen in the Case of those that die of Famine: for take the soundest Person, and deprive him of all liquid and solid Aliment, the Salts become continually more and more acrimonious; till at length a Fever, Delirium, *&c.* are brought on by their great Irritation, which soon ends in universal Putrefac-

* *Cap.* iii. *De variolarum curationibus.*

tion and Death.—You may see how this Putrescence of Humors advances by taking a *healthy Nurse,* whose Milk, for some Hours after eating, is white, thin, sweet, and grateful; let her fast for sixteen or eighteen Hours, it becomes thick, yellow, salt, and disagreeable: Let her further abstain for some few Hours longer, it turns of a much deeper yellow, nauseous, and even stinking; and all this much more so, if she happens to labour under a Fever, a bloody Kind of Matter issuing instead of Milk.—If this happens to the most acescent and sweetest Humor of the Body, what think you happens to the Bile, Lymph, *&c.*

Where the Heat and Attrition of the Blood are very considerable, its Putrefaction advances surprisingly fast. It appears from* *Boerhaave's* Experiment on a Dog, shut up in a hot Sugar-baker's Stove, that the whole Mass of Humors was corrupted to so high a Degree, in a few Minutes, as to give off an insupportable Stench; and so dissolved, that the very *Saliva* became *bloody*; and so horribly offensive, as to throw a strong Man, concerned in the Experiment, into Faintings.

The animal Humors naturally run into Dissolution and Putrefaction, unless prevented and corrected by daily Supplies of *acescent Aliment*; a Diet merely of Flesh, Fish, Spices, and Water, will very soon bring on a putrid Fever.—*Bread* is not only the *Staff of Life,* as Nourishment, but as it also corrects, by its acescent Quality, the rank Juices of animal Food.—The *Spanish* and *French Prisoners here,* by eating unusual and immoderate Quantities of Flesh, brought on such dangerous Fevers as carried off vast Numbers of them.—They were so fond of it, that they died, as it were, with Flesh in their Mouths frequently.

But thus much for the Generation of *alcalescent Acrimony* in the Blood: Let me add, that it seems to appear, from what is above said, that, in some Cases, the animal Salts are rendered actually alcaline, volatile, corrosive, and destructive of the Blood-gloubles, as well as the *minima Vascula*, while even Life subsists.—When the animal Oils are also highly exalted and rancid, they unite with these Salts, and make a most destructive dissolving *Sapo*, much of the Nature of putrid Bile, which corrodes and dissolves all the Principles of Life.

Now, as, on the one Hand, an *acrimonious State* of Blood may be complicated with too tense rigid Fibres, and an *inflammatory*

* *Vide Boerhaavii Chem. Cap. de Igne, Experiment* xx. *Coroll.* 16.

Lentor; so, on the other, it may consist with a *thin dissolved State* of Blood and *weak lax Fibres.*

Let us put Contagion for Acrimony, (for it acts in a like Manner, and eventually proves so) and we have the Cases very justly exemplified in the Small-pox: Where the Disease is sometimes attended with a very viscid State of Blood, high inflammatory Fever, violent acute Pains, peripneumonic Symptoms, Phrenzy and the like: Sometimes on the contrary with a weak, dissolved Blood, a low slow Pulse, or a weak and quick one, nervous Symptoms, thin crude Urine, various and profuse Hæmorrhages, little or no Pain, Swelling, Soreness, or the like. In the former Case the Fever runs too high, and burns up the Patient; in the latter there is not Fever enough to make a compleat Protrusion and Maturation of the Pustules, but they remain sessile, crude and Undigested; whence at last the whole Mass of Blood runs into a putrid corrosive *Ichor*, or a gangrenous *Sanies.*

Take another View of this Matter.—I have many Times known *pulmonic*, or *pleuro-peripneumonic* Fevers attack Persons of a very thin acrid State of Blood, which have been attended with a very considerable Degree of Inflammation.—This happens very frequently to scorbutic seafaring Persons.

In the Years 1740 and 1745, Abundance of People were seized with Shivering, then great Heats, Fever and Difficulty of Breathing, importunate laborious Coughs, very acute darting Pains of the Breasts, Sides and Back, and frequently also in the Head and Temples. They had oftentimes a very quick, hard Pulse, but *concentrated* as it were; the Breath was very hot and offensive, and the Matter they expectorated was sometimes thin and crude, and sometimes as yellow as Saffron; but much more commonly a thin, gleety bloody Matter, frequently very foetid, and sometimes so acrid as to cause a great Hoarseness, and Soreness of the Wind-pipe and Throat, and sometimes Excoriations of those Parts. The Blood drawn from them was either of a darkish livid Colour, covered over with a lead-coloured or greenish thin Film, or sometimes qutie florid (particularly on the first Bleeding) but of a loose, soft Consistence when cold; the specious Appearance often surprising the Surgeon, or Apothecary, who expected quite another Appearance of the Blood, considering the Symptoms. However in many of these Fevers, the Blood drawn was covered over with a pretty thick tough Coat, not of a whitish yellow Colour, as usual in common pleuritic or pleuro-peripneumonic Blood, but of a Colour approaching to that of a *Cornelian Stone,* or a little more dilute than that of the common Jelly of *red Currants.*—This Colour of the *Buff* on Blood I constantly observe to be of ill Omen: I conjecture because it indicates both a great Glutinosity, and also a very great Quantity of acrid Salts in the Blood, which break its Globules, and put it into a putrid dissolving State; for this Appearance seems to arise from the broken Globules inviscated by the inflammatory Size. If a Portion of volatile-alcali Salt be mixed with the Blood of a Person in a high Pleurisy, as it runs off from the Vein, the upper Part of the *Crassamentum* will greatly resemble that of the Blood, which I have just mentioned: And it is further remarkable, that the *Serum* of such Kind of Blood hath very often a *bloody Tinge,* almost as high as *Burgundy Wine;* and so indeed frequently had the *Serum* of the other Kinds of Blood, tho' many Times it appeared only of a turbid yellow Colour. The Urine was commonly very high, and sometimes dark-coloured with a Kind of lead-coloured Sediment; it was generally rendered in small Quantities. Faint, uncertain, partial Sweats often attended, particularly about the Face and Head; although many Times, towards the fatal Period, they were very profuse and colliquative. Livid, or black Spots frequently appeared about the State of the Disease, and I think seldom, or never failed of being the certain Harbingers of Death. The black and brown Thrush, which also sometimes broke out towards the Close, were not of a much more favourable Prognostic. But an universal, burning, itching, Rash sometimes terminated the Fever; and sometimes it ended in an Eruption of very large, angry, ulcerating Pustules on the Neck, Shoulders and Arms, but more especially about the Nose and Lips.

But of this Kind of peripneumonic Fever more hereafter, with the Method of treating it.—I shall only at present take Notice, that at the same Time when this malignant Peripneumony, if I may so call it, reigned in *Plymouth,* and its Neighbourhood, Pleurisies, Peripneumonies, and Pleuro-peripneumonies were every-where epidemic, and generally of the true inflammatory Kind, arising from the cold dry northerly and easterly Winds, which had for a long Time prevailed.—In these the Blood was very dense and sizy, and most commonly covered over with a very thick, white, or yellowish Buff; and the Sick bore the Loss of Blood well and to Advantage, even to forty Ounces, or upwards sometimes: Whereas the Blood, in the *malignant pulmonic Fever, was as I have above described it;*

and, when it was considerably buffy, it had the *above-mentioned Appearance,* and the Patients often sunk surprisingly after the first or second Bleeding; sometimes indeed to my great Concern and Astonishment; when, from the hard Pulse, great Load at Breast, pungent Pain of the Side, and Severity of the Cough, I thought I had sufficient Warranty for advising it.—Besides, tho' these latter expectorated pretty large Quantities of crude and thin, or more frequently of a gleety bloody Matter, they were not at all relieved; whereas when the *former* spit off largely and freely, it was of the highest Advantage.

Now I must further take Notice, that, *cotemporary with both these Disorders a contagious, putrid, petechial fever* was very rife in and about this *Town*; especially among the Sailors and Prisoners, and those that were very conversant with them; and it was chiefly among those Sorts of Persons, that the *malignant pulmonic Fever* raged.—So that this seemed to be a Complication of the common inflammatory Peripneumony with the contagious petechial Fever: the *contagious Effluvia* acting on the Blood in the Manner of *acrimonious Salts,* and destroying its *Crasis.*—It is certain we frequently meet with Peripneumonies of this Kind, merely from the sharp acrid State of the Humors of those that are seized with them.

Now these are Fevers, in which an inflammatory Lentor is complicated with a greater Degree of Acrimony, or blended with a Kind of poisonous dissolving *Effluvia.*—But we often meet with others, in which a very high Acrimony of the Humors is combined with a *too lax State* of the Vessels, and too *loosely compacted Blood-globules;* which is the Case very commonly in petechial Fevers, especially such as are attended with Hæmorrhages.

I here beg leave to give the History of such an one, which I think was the severest, that ever any Person suffered under, who survived the Disease:—And the rather, as I shall specify the Method of his Cure; which not only in his Case, but in several others of the like Nature, tho' not Degree, I have experienced to be highly beneficial; and which, I am persuaded, is the only successful Course that can be used in them, however different it may seem from the common Practice.

An eminent Surgeon of a neighbouring Town, of a thin and somewhat tender Constitution, but constantly used to Action and Exercise, and frequently subject to Fevers, and scorbutic Rheumatisms, from taking Cold, *&c.* in *October* 1741, fell into a Kind of slow Fever, attended with slight Rigors, Frequent Flushes of Heat, a quick weak Pulse, Loss of Strength and Appetite, with a great Load at his Breast, and a heavy Sort of Respiration.—Notwithstanding this, he continued in his Business, constantly riding, and fatiguing himself for some four or five Days after this Seizure.—I met him at a Gentleman's House, who was my Patient; and finding him as above, and that his Breath was, even then, very offensive, I earnestly desired him to take timely and due Care of himself.—Two Days after, he, being at a Gentleman's in the Neighbourhood, was taken all on a sudden with a very great Faintness, and fell off his Chair: Upon lifting him up the Company observed several livid and violet-coloured Spots on his Arms and Neck. It was with very great Difficulty they got him Home, tho' but two or three Miles Distance, he very frequently fainting by the Way.—The Disorder encreased every Moment, he had a vast Languor with Pain and extream Oppression on the Præcordia, and a perpetual Sighing:—his Breath now stank abominably, and a foetid bloody Matter leaked continually from his Gums, and thousands of livid, violet and black Spots appeared all over his Body, on the Trunk, as well as the Limbs.

He was bled to about ℥xii from his Arm, but this gave him no Manner of Relief, the Oppression, Sighing, Fainting, and Anxiety continuing as bad as ever, nay rather encreasing;—a violent Hæmorrhage also broke forth from his Nose; which continuing from both Nostrils, he was bled again to ℥x about twelve Hours after the former Bleeding:—neither did this give him any Relief, but encreased his Weakness considerably, and he continued as anxious, restless, and oppressed as ever, without even the least Sleep. The Blood now not only issued from his Gums and Nose, but he also coughed up Blood.—Indeed the Bleeding from his Nose had ceased somewhat, but it encreased from his Gums, and in a surprising Manner. Blood now likewise dropped, tho' slowly, from the Caruncle of one of his Eyes; and several livid Pustules on his Tongue, and withinside his Lips, broke, and discharged a bloody, thin Matter very copiously.

The Hæmorrhage being somewhat restrained, a bloody Dysentery came on with severe Gripes, and excessive Faintness, and he was still exceeding restless and very feverish: his Pulse now intermitted every sixth or eighth Pulsation, and then fluttered on again vastly quick; he had likewise a constant *Tremor* and *Subsultus.*—The Hæmorrhage all this while continued from one Part or other, and when stopped at one Place forthwith burst out at another; so that his Urine now seemed tinged with Blood, being very dark-coloured, nay almost black. Soon after he was bled the second Time, I was sent for, and hastened to him.—I found him in the Manner described, under an inexpressible Anxiety, yet quite free from a Delirium, though he had no Manner of Sleep for several Days and Nights: His Tongue was vastly black, and his Breath so insufferably stinking, that it was greatly offensive even at a considerable Distance; and his Stools were so horribly nauseous and foetid, that the very Nurses fell into Vomitings and Faintness in carrying them off.

I found that neither of the Portions of the Blood that had been drawn (not even the first) had separated into *Crassamentum* and *Serum* as usual, tho' the former had stood so many Hours; but continued as it were half coagulated, and of a bluish livid Colour on the Top:—it was most easily divided by the slightest Touch, and seemed a *purulent Sanies* rather than Blood, with a Kind of a *sooty Powder* at Bottom. His Hæmorrhage still continued, especially from the Tongue, Lips, and Gums, with a perpetual Dripping of thin bloody Ichor from his Nose; so that he was reduced to an extream Degree of Weakness, with never ceasing Tremblings, *Subsultus Tendinum,* and almost continual Faintings.

What was to be done in this dreadful Case? Would the hot, alexipharmac, volatile Cordials and Blisters have served him, as some might have imagined, considering his extream Weakness, Faintings, Load on the Præcordia, Tremblings, *&c?* But would they not have been certainly *deleterious,* would they not have certainly killed him? as they would have added to the stimulating Acrimony, encreased the Fever, and further destroyed the *Crasis* of the Blood, already nearly quite dissolved, and reduced to a Kind of *putrid Gore.*

I took it in this View, and, as I had experimentally and repeatedly known the great Use of the *Bark** in preventing and stopping the Advance of Gangrenes, I gave him frequently of it in small Doses with *Elixir Vitrioli,* premising a small Quantity of *Rhubarb.* —Besides this he drank Tincture of Roses, with Cinnamon Water, made very acid, and also a Decoction of *Sevil* Orange Rind, red Roses, Cinnamon, and a little *Japon* Earth (as it is called) well

*** Besides I had formerly given the Bark with Success in the malignant petechial Fever of 1735:** ***Vid. Obs. de Aere et Morb. Epidem. Mense Maio.***

acidulated: Claret, and red Port, with about half Water, he drank at Pleasure.—As the *Bark* sat easy with him, I continued its Use, and encreased its Quantity, giving with it some *Confect. Fracast. sine melle* to restrain the dysenteric Flux;—and yet I now and then interposed a small Dose of *Rhubarb*, to carry off any bloody, bilious, or sanious Matter that might be lodged in, or leak into the Intestines. In the mean Time I ordered him to be frequently supported with Rice, Panado, Sago, Jellies of Harts-horn well acidulated. Toast out of Claret, or red Port Wine; and I directed Fomentations of Aromatics and Astringents, boiled in red Wine, to be frequently applied to the whole Abdomen.

By this Method, steadily persisted in, was this poor Gentleman, thro' divine Goodness, raised from a State of universal Rottenness, as it were, to perfect Health: Not but that, for a very considerable Time after his Fever was quite gone off, he continued extreamly weak; and even after he was capable of walking abroad, the Hæmorrhage from his Nose would return on the least Occasion, his Gums would bleed on the slightest Rubbing, and his Breath continued very offensive for a long Time.—By the further Use of the *Cortex, Elix. Vitrioli,* &c. this also intirely ceased:—But his Legs and Feet continued very much swoln for a much longer Time, and his Flesh all over the whole Body remained exceeding soft, tender, and sore, scarce bearing the least Touch.—Rhabarbarate Purges, easy stomachic Chalybeates, Elixir of Vitriol, *Pyrmont* Water with proper Diuretics, and gentle regular Exercise at length carried off all those Symptoms; and in about two or three Months he recovered a good State of Health, which he still enjoys.

I met with several of these petechial Fevers, with Hæmorrhages in the Summer and Autumn of 1745; particularly a Gentlewoman, of *Anthony* near *Plymouth*, was seized with such a Fever, with Symptoms nearly resembling those in the above-mentioned Case, tho' not in so high a Degree.—She fell into an immense Discharge from the *Uterus*, tho' out of Season, after a very profuse Hæmorrhage from the Nose; she bled also from the Gums, and at last had a bloody Dysentery: She had a strong Phrenzy before the Bleeding from the Nose came on, and had a vast Number of purple and black Spots all over her Body, some as large, at least, as a Silver Penny.—I treated her exactly in the Manner aforesaid, and she happily recovered; tho' her Legs were greatly swoln after it, and she continued in a long State of Weakness.—She was twice bled before I saw her;—

the first Blood I saw not, but Mr. *Freke*, her Surgeon, told me it was very Florid and rich (as he called it) but very soft, and gave off a very small Quantity of a reddish *Serum*: I saw the second, which was of a very dark black Colour, covered with a very thin, tender, greenish Skin.—Her Urine, during the whole Time of the Fever almost, was like white Wine, or Cyder, that stands long exposed to the Air, and turns black; at length however a Kind of a dark coloured mealy Sediment was deposited.

The Fever, which attends Gangrenes, is commonly of this Kind, corrupting and dissolving the Blood; the sanious Matter of the gangrened Part, being resorbed into the Mass of Blood, produces an universal gangrenous Disposition in the Humors, and dissolves the sound red Globules; whence Spots, Hæmorrhages, black Tongues, Delirium, *&c.* supervene. *Celsus** justly observes that an acute Fever, Delirium, great Thirst, and stinking Breath, accompany a Gangrene; all Signs of Corruption of the Blood and high Acrimony. —I will instance but in one Case, which, I think, is pretty uncommon in several Circumstances.

Mrs. *Elisabeth S—th* of St. *Germains in Cornwall*, about twenty-five, of a weak Constitution and bad Habit of Body, who never had any regular *Catamenia*, was taken at the latter End of *May*, 1742, with a Pain in the right Foot near the Toes, and with a *Torpor* all over the Leg; which hourly encreasing, she sent for Mr. *Dyer*, an ingenious Surgeon of *Looe*, who rubbed the Part with camphorated Spirit of Wine, and gave her some nervous and cordial Medicines.—This having no Effect, he fomented with a very warm aromatic Decoction, applying the *Magma* with Spirits, Theriaca, *&c.* to the Leg and Foot; notwithstanding which the Parts grew soon discoloured, cold and quite insensible.—When I came, I ordered the Parts to be scarified, and that deeply, but not the least Blood issued, only a few Drops of quite black Blood here and there slowly rose up, of the Bigness of a Pea;—the Skin and Flesh looked as if the Leg had been cut off for some Days, tho' this was but in the Forenoon of the *fourth Day* from the very first Seizure.—There were no Vesications, nor did the Scarifications afterwards emit the least Stench, Matter, or *Sanies.*—I immediately ordered her the *Bark* with *Elixir Vitriol. Confect. Ralegh.* and a warm acidulated Julep, which she took freely, as she was vastly faint.—A violent Pain seized her in the Afternoon in her right Thigh and Groin, and

* *Lib. V. Cap.* 26.

forthwith a Fever, severe Gripings, and a bloody Flux, came on, which presently reduced her to the utmost Degree of Weakness, with perpetual Faintings and Agonies.

The ensuing Night she grew very delirious, her Tongue became quite black and faultering her Pulse exceeding quick, weak and fluttering, with continual Catchings of the Tendons and Tremors.—As the *Cortex* did not sit well, but ran down, I gave her a strong Tincture of it with *Decoct. Fracastor. Elix. Vitriol.* &c. which had a much better Effect.

In this miserable Condition she continued for three or four Days, every one about her hourly expecting her Death; however the *Sphacelation* did not advance, and never appeared above the Knee, tho' a very vehement Pain affected the whole Thigh, and seemed chiefly in the *Periosteum* of the Bone.—At length there appeared a dark, livid *Streak* or *Line* all round the Limb, immediately under the Knee, and pointed out where Nature was disposed to separate the dead Part from the living. This Tendency to Separation became every Day more and more visible, and the Surgeon used all proper Means to promote it: For whatever Foundation there might have been for an *Amputation,* neither she, nor her Friends, would admit of it.—In these deplorable Circumstances (the dead Part of the Limb daily rotting off from the sound) she continued till *July* the 14th; when the Surgeon, finding the *Slough* cast off, and a Separation at the Joint almost perfectly made, took off with a Knife the dead Leg from the sound Thigh, at the *very Articulation,* with very little Pain, without her Consent, and almost without her Knowledge of it, when it was done.—Soon after this she daily recovered, and by proper Diet, and Medicines, was in a little Time restored to a tolerable State of Health.

CHAP. VI.

Of the Difference between a slow nervous, and a putrid malignant Fever.

I cannot conclude this Essay on Fevers, without taking Notice of the very great Difference there is between the *putrid malignant,* and the *slow nervous Fever*; the Want of which Distinction, I am fully persuaded, hath been often productive of no small Errors in Practice, as they resemble one another in some Respects, tho' very essentially different in others.—And this I the rather do now, as I have not sufficiently noted the Difference in my *Dissertation de Febribus lentis & nervosis.*—Nor do I know of any Author, that hath done it explicitly, besides Dr. *Langrish* in his *Modern Theory and Practice.*

By what hath been said above, I think, it evidently appears, that in putrid malignant and petechial Fevers the *Blood, peculiarly so called,* is affected; whereas the slow nervous Fevers seem to have their Seat chiefly in the *lymphatic and nervous Juices.* Corruption of the Humors and Dissolution of the Blood are in a high Degree observable in the former; but the slow nervous Fever frequently runs on to a great Length of Time, without any considerable Signs of Putrefaction.

Besides, these two different Kinds of Fevers may be artificially produced, if I may so speak, by two very different Kinds of Diet, Regimen, *&c.* and is too often actually effected. The hot, acrid, saline, volatile and spicy Food, and Medicines, very hot Air, *&c.* will produce a putrid malignant:—On the contrary, cold, watery, slimy, mucilaginous Things, as Cucumbers, Melons, crude trashy Fruit, vapid Liquors, damp cold Air, *&c.* bring on slow nervous Fevers.

Could we suppose both the one and the other to arise from Contagion, (which is commonly the Case in pestilential and petechial Fevers, and may sometimes be so in the slow nervous) I should liken the Action of the *morbific Effluvia* in the former, to that of the Poison of a Viper, which immediately affects and destroys the Texture of the Blood-globules, and brings on a very speedy Corruption:—But in the latter to the *Virus* of a mad Dog, which works but slowly, and seems primarily to affect the *Lymph,* and *Succus nervosus,* and manifests no Signs of Putridity, at least till the very Close of the Tragedy.

Now as these two Fevers have a very different Origin, they cannot but shew their Effects in different Symptoms, and require a very different Method of Cure;—and yet, I am very sensible, the one may be, and very often is, blended with the other; I mean, that a very acrimonious State of Blood may subsist under a very weak relaxed System of Vessels, and may not shew itself with so much Violence, as if the moving Powers and Vessels were more strong and elastic, and much more susceptive of the *Stimulus* of the morbid, acrimonious Salts, *&c.* and of Course more slow in its Progress, tho' perhaps equally fatal.—The different antecedent State of the Fibres, and Powers of Nature, where Contagion is the proximate Cause of the Disease, doth undoubtedly alter the Nature of the subsequent Fever very greatly.—By carefully describing both these Fevers, their Nature and Difference will more fully appear.

CHAP. VII.

Of the slow nervous Fever.

I Begin with a Description of the slow nervous Fever, which hath been very exactly taken from too many, who have fallen Victims to this insidious and dangerous Enemy.

The Patient at first grows somewhat listless, and feels slight Chills and Shudders, with uncertain sudden Flushes of Heat, and a Kind of Weariness all over, like what is felt after great Fatigue: This is always attended with a Sort of Heaviness and Dejection of Spirit, and more or less of a Load, Pain, or Giddiness of the Head; a *Nausea* and Disrelish of every Thing soon follows, without any considerable Thirst, but frequently with urging to Vomit, tho' little but insipid Phlegm is brought up.

Tho' a Kind of lucid Interval of several Hours sometimes intervenes, yet the Symptoms return with Aggravation, especially towards Night: The Head grows more heavy, or giddy, the Heats greater, the Pulse quicker, but weak, with an oppressive Kind of Breathing.—A great *Torpor*, or obtuse Pain and Coldness affects the hinder Part of the Head frequently, and oftentimes a heavy Pain is felt on the Top all along the *coronary Suture*; this, and that of the back part of the Head, generally attend nervous Fevers, and are commonly succeeded by some Degree of a Delirium.

In this Condition the Patient often continues for five or six Days, with a heavy pale sunk Countenance, seeming not very sick, and yet far from being well; restless, anxious, and commonly quite void of Sleep, tho' sometimes very drowsy and heavy: but although he appears to those about him actually to sleep, he is utterly insensible of it, and denies that he doth so.

The Pulse, during all this Time, is quick, weak and unequal, sometimes fluttering, and sometimes for a few Minutes slow, nay intermitting; and then, with a sudden Flush in the Face,—immediately very quick, and perhaps soon after surprisingly calm and equal; and thus alternately.—The Heats and Chills are as uncertain and unequal, sometimes a sudden Colour and Glow in the Cheeks, while the Tip of the Nose and Ears is cold, and the Forehead at the same Time in a cold dewy Sweat.—Nay it is very common, that a high Colour and Heat appear in the Face, when the Extremities are quite cold.

The Urine is commonly pale, and often limpid, frequently of a Whey-colour, or like vapid Small-beer in which there is either no Manner of Sediment, or a Kind of loose Matter, like Bran, irregularly scattered up and down in it.—The Tongue, at the Begining, is seldom or never dry or discoloured, but sometimes covered with a thin whitish *Mucus*;—at length indeed it often appears very dry, red, and chapped, or of the Colour of Pomegranate Rind; but this mostly at the State, or Close of the Disease: yet, however dry the Tongue and Lips seem, the Patient scarce ever complains of Thirst, tho' sometimes of a Heat in the Tongue.

About the seventh or eighth Day the Giddiness, Pain, or Heaviness of the Head, become much greater, with a constant Noise in it, or *Tinnitus Aurium*, which is very disturbing to the Sick, and frequently brings on a Delirium. The Load on the Præcordia, Anxiety and Faintness grow much more urgent, and they often fall into an actual *Deliquium*; especially if they attempt to sit up; Coldish Sweats suddenly come on in the Forehead, and on the Backs of the Hands (tho' at the same Time there is too much Heat in the Cheeks and the Palms) and as suddenly go off.—If the Urine now grows more pale and limpid, and Delitum is certainly to be expected with universal Tremors and *Subsultus Tendinum*; the Delirium is seldom violent, but as it were a Confusion of Thought and Action, muttering continually to themselves, and faultering in their Speech: Sometimes they awake only in a Hurry and Confusion, and presently recollect themselves, but forthwith fall into a muttering, dozy State again.

The Tongue grows often very dry at the State, especially in its middle Part, with a yellowish List on each Side, and it trembles greatly when the Sick attempt to put it out.—When the Tongue at this Time grows more moist, and a copious Spitting comes on, it is always a very good Sign:—But where a Difficulty of swallowing, continual *Gulping,* or *Choaking* in the Throat supervene, it is a very dangerous Symptom, especially if attended with any Degree of a *Singultus.*

Frequently profuse Sweats pour forth all at once about the ninth, tenth, or twelfth Day, commonly coldish and clammy on the Extremities: oftentimes very thin Stools are discharged; both the one and the other are generally colliquative and very weakening.—However a warm Moisture of the Skin is generally salutary, and a gentle Diarrhœa frequently carries off the Delirium and comatose Disposition.

Now Nature sinks apace, the Extremities grow cold, the Nails pale or livid, the Pulse may be said to tremble and flutter rather than to beat, the Vibrations being so exceeding weak and quick, that they can scarce be distinguished; tho' sometimes they creep on surprisingly slow, and very frequently intermit. The Sick become quite insensible and stupid, scarce affected with the loudest Noise, or the strongest Light; tho' at the Begining strangely susceptive of the Impressions of either. The Delirium now ends in a profound *Coma,* and that soon in eternal Sleep.—The Stools, Urine, and Tears run off involuntarily, and denounce a speedy Dissolution, as the vast Tremblings and Twitching of the Nerves and Tendons are Preludes to a general Convulsion, which at once snaps off the Thread of Life.—In one or other of these Ways are the Sick carried off, after having languished on for fourteen, eighteen, or twenty Days; nay, sometimes much longer.

All Persons grow deaf and stupid towards the End of the Disease (some extreamly deaf) tho' too quick and apprehensive at the Begining, insomuch that the least Noise, or Light, greatly offended them.—Many, from their immoderate Fears, seem to hurry themselves out of Life, where little Danger was apparent at the Begining; nay several will not suffer themselves to sleep, from a vain Fear of dozing quite away; and others from the vast Hurry, Anxiety, and Confusion, they are sensible of in it, or at their awaking.—Where the Deafness ends in an Impostume of the Ear, it is generally a good Symptom; and so it is also when a *Parotis* suppurates, or a large pustular angry Eruption breaks out about the Lips and Nose.

This is a Description, (tedious indeed, but pretty exact) of the slow nervous Fever in its most aggravated Circumstances: Wherein I have laid down the Symptoms in the Order in which they naturally come on;—and this I think should be always observed in describing any Disease.—It most commonly attacks persons of weak Nerves, a lax Habit of Body, and a poor thin Blood; those who have suffered great Evacuations, a long Dejection of Spirits, immoderate Watchings, Studies, Fatigue, and the like; and also those, who have used much crude unwholesome Food, vapid impure Drinks, or who have been confined long in damp, foul air; that have broken the Vigor of their Constitutions by Salivations, too frequent Purging, immoderate Venery, *&c.*—Whence I think it is evident, this Disease arises from a too relaxed State of the Solids, a poor weak Blood, and a *Lentor and Vapidity of the lymphatic and nervous Juices:*—The very Method of Cure shews this, which consists in mild, stimulating, attenuating, and Proper Cordial, strengthening Diet and Medicines.—*Hippocrates* somewhere notes, that the successful Method of Cure shews the Nature of the Disease.

Let us now therefore endeavour to shew the properest Method of curing this Fever.

It was another Maxim of the great *Hippocrates*, that whoever knows the Nature of the Disease, knows the Method of Cure*.—It is at least the indispensable Duty of every Physician, before he prescribes for his Patient, to consider well his Constitution, and the Nature of his Disease; for as *Celsus* elegantly says, *Æstimatio causæ sæpe morbum solvit*†.—And this is in no Case more necessary than in Fevers, in which the Time is short, and Experiments dangerous: Where the Disorder doth not attack with great Violence, it is better to wait a little, and observe the Motions of Nature, than be too precipitant.—But it is rare, that Physicians are called in at the very Begining of slow Fevers: Indeed they are often too far advanced, 'ere they are consulted.

From the History of the slow nervous Fever I think it is very evident, that no great Evacuations are proper (especially Bleeding) particularly in Persons of originally weak and lax Constitutions, who are by far the most subject to it.—I have known a common Purge, injudiciously given at the Begining of this Fever, immediately followed by surprising Languors, *Syncope*, and a large Train of other ill Symptoms: However it may be necessary sometimes, even at the Begining, to cleanse the *primæ Viæ*, by a gentle Puke, a little *Rhubarb, Manna, &c;* if you give any Thing *drastic*, be assured

* *Lib. de Arte sub sinem.*

† *Celsi Præsat. sub sinem.*

your Patient will rue for it, and you will repent it.—And here I cannot but observe, that a mild Vomit may be given with much less Ruffle to Nature than a common Purge, and indeed is useful, nay necessary, where Nausea, Load and Sickness at Stomach are urgent; which frequently happen at the Attack of this Fever:—Clysters of Milk, Sugar, and Salt, may be injected with Safety and Advantage every second or third Day, if Nature wants to be prompted to stool.

The temperate, cordial, diaphoretic Medicines are certainly most proper in these Fevers; and a well regulated, supporting, diluting Diet is necessary: The latter of itself, judiciously managed, will go a great Way in the Cure, especially assisted by well timed and well applied Blisters, and a due Care to keep the Patient as quiet as possible, both in Body and Mind. But it should be noted, that any strong *Opiates* are commonly very pernicious, however Want of Sleep and great Restlessness may seem to demand them.—Mild Diaphoretics, as *Pulv. Contrayeru. comp.* with a little Castor and Saffron, and small Quantities of *Theriac. Andromachi*, or *Elixir Paregoricum*, have much better Effects: which, by raising a gentle easy Sweat, or at least a plentiful Perspiration, calm the Hurry and Tumult of the Blood and Spirits, whence soft refreshing Slumber succeeds. Where the Confusion and Dejection of Spirits are very considerable, *Galbanum* or *Silphium*, with a little Camphire, should be added; and Blisters should be forthwith applied to the Neck, *Occiput*, or behind the Ears: and during all this a free Use of thin Wine-whey, some pleasant Ptisan, or Gruel, with a little soft Wine, must be indulged. Indeed the Patients, in this Case, should drink frequently: though such Quantities may not be necessary as in the ardent, or even putrid malignant Fevers; yet they should be sufficient to carry on the Work of Dilution, support the Sweats, and supply the Blood with fresh and wholesome Fluids, in lieu of the vapid, acrid *Latex*, that is continually passing off.—And I think in this View a thin Chicken Broth also is of Service, both as Food and Physic, especially towards the Decline of the Disorder; and for the same Reason thin Jellies of Hart's-horn, Sago, Panado, are useful, adding a little Wine to them, and the Juice of Sevile Orange, or Lemon.

It is observable, the Sick are never so easy, as whilst they are in a gentle easy Sweat; for this soon removes the Exacerbations of Heat, Hurry, *&c.* —But profuse Sweats should never be encouraged, much less attempted by very strong heating Medicines, volatile alcalious Salts, Spirits, *&c*; especially in the Begining, or Advance of the Fever; for they too much exhaust the *Liquidum vitale*, and are followed by a vast Dejection of Spirits, Tremors, Startings of the Tendons, and sometimes end in *Rigors*, cold clammy Sweats, *Syncope*, or a comatose Disposition.—Sometimes irregular, partial Heats and Flushes succeed, with great Anxiety, Restlessness, Delirium, Difficulty of Breathing, and a vast Load and Oppression on the *Præcordia*; so as to incline the less cautious Observer to think there may be something peripneumonic in it:—but even here beware of Bleeding, for you will find the Pulse very small and unequal, though very quick: Not only the Weakness and Fluttering of the Pulse contraindicate Bleeding, but also the pale, watery, limpid Urine, which is commonly attendant. These Symptoms denote the Load, Anxiety, and Oppression on the *Præcordia* to be from the nervous *Orgasm*, not from a peripneumonic Obstruction, or Inflammation: The Breathing in this Case, though thick and laborious, is not hot, but a Kind of a sighing, or sobbing Respiration, nor is there many Times any Kind of Cough concomitant; so that this is really from some Degree of Spasm on the Vitals, not from Inflammation.—And this is very manifest in hysteric Paroxysms.

Here therefore the nervous cordial Medicines are indicated, and Blisters to the Thighs, Legs, or Arms.— I commonly use the following *Bolus* and *Saline Draught*.

℞ *Pulv. Contrayerv. c. gr.* xv.* *Croc. Anglic. gr.* iii. *Confect. Ralegh.* ℈i. *Syr. Croci q. s. m. f. Bolus.*

℞ *Sal. C.C.* ℈ss. *Succ. Limon.* ʒiii. *Aq. alexet. simpl.* ℥iss.*m. peractâ effervescentiâ adde Sp. Lavend. c. Syr. Croci ana* ʒiss. *m. f. Haust.*

These, or the like, I order every 5th, 6th, or 8th Hour, and a temperate cordial Julep; *Spiritus volatilis aromat.* or *fœtidus* may be now and then given out of thin Wine, or Cyder-whey, or, which is in many Cases better, out of thin Mustard-whey; which, without any more pompous *Apparatus*, is not a contemptible Medicine, especially for the Poor. These gently stimulate the torpid Vessels, and raise their oscillatory Powers; they attenuate the Humors and dilute them, and by these Means promote easy relieving Sweats, which soon carry off the *Erethism*, as the Ancients called it.—The Saline

* *When vast Tremors and Subsultus Tendinum come on, I use Musk* ℈ss *instead of the* Pulv. Contrayerv. *c. with great* Success.

Draught, prepared as above, is much more apt to pass by the Pores of the Skin than when made with Salt of Wormwood, which rather moves through the urinary Passages.—When I assert, from repeated Experience, the Use of the above described Draught in asthmatic Cases, any one may easily judge of its Efficacy in these.

But to return, this Difficulty of Breathing, Anxiety and Oppression, many Times precede a *miliary Eruption*, which often appears the seventh, ninth, or eleventh Day of this Fever, and sometimes later:—Indeed great Anxiety and Oppression on the *Præcordia* always precede pustular Eruptions of any Kind, in all Sorts of Fevers.—Every one must know how ill-timed and improper Bleeding would be on such an Occasion, when the greatest Care should be taken not to retard Nature's Operation in this particular, which is many Times compleatly critical: On the contrary it should be promoted by soft, easy Cordials, proper Diluents and the like; and to these sometimes a little *Theriaca Andromachi*, or *Elixir Asthmaticum*, should be added; which not only tend to calm the universal Uneasiness commonly complained of, but also very effectually promote a *Diaphoresis*, or breathing kindly Sweats, with which the miliary Eruptions freely and easily advance.

But however advantageous these commonly are, profuse Sweats are seldom or never so, even though attended with a very large Eruption; for I have known two or three Crops of miliary Pustules succeed one another, and large Sweats, long continued, with no Manner of Relief to the Patients; nay of very great Detriment, as they reduced them to an extream Degree of Weakness.—In Truth these large Sweats are much more commonly *symptomatical* than critical, and the consequent Eruption is very often the mere *Symptom* of a *Symptom*; for the miliary Glands of the Skin appear very turgid, and *mimic a Rash* upon profuse Sweating, even in the most healthy.

In such profuse, colliquative Sweats, I have very frequently given a little generous red Wine, (diluted somewhat, if necessary) with the greatest Advantage; it presently moderating the Sweat, supporting the Patient, and keeping up also the miliary *Papulæ*, if they happen likewise to attend.—*Celsus* advises *Vinum austerum meraculum in morbo cardiaco**, which I take to have been a Species of nervous Fever with colliquative Sweats.—Towards the Decline of the Fever, where the Sweats are abundant and weakening, I moreover give

* *Lib. III. Cap. 19.*

small Doses of the Tincture of the Bark with Saffron and Snake Root, hereafter described, interposing now and then a Dose of Rhubarb to carry off the putrid *Colluvies,* in the first Passages; which withal makes the *Remissions,* or *Intermissions,* which frequently happen in the Decline of nervous Fevers, more distinct and manifest, and gives a fairer Opportunity for Preparations of the *Bark.*—I generally give it, about this Time, out of the saline Draughts made with Salt of Wormwood and Juice of Lemons, which makes them much more effectual. I am persuaded this Method will shorten these Fevers, even those with miliary Eruptions, which too often run on to an exceeding great Length, and are frequently attended with dangerous Relapses.—I have more than once known Patients sink under this Fever, after having been kept in a sweating Method for five or six Weeks together, and after having gone thro' three or four successive Crops of miliary Eruptions (as they were called) they all the while melting away, and weltering in their own Sweat, and the Bed rotting under them.

Though a gentle Diarrhœa is sometimes of manifest Service towards the End of this Fever, crude, thin, colliquative Stools are very far from being so, but sink the Sick surprisingly fast: Where they are livid, or of a Kind of lead Colour, whatever be the Consistence, it is a dangerous Appearance.

There is no Evacuation of a more favourable Portent than a pretty free Salivation, without *Aphthæ*; where this happens, with a kindly Moisture of the Skin, I never despair of my Patient, however weak and stupid he may seem:—Indeed the Deafness many Times makes the Sick, at the Close of the Distemper, appear much less sensible than they really are; not but that many, under these Circumstances, escaping the Grave, degenerate into mere Idiots.

Under any of these Evacuations plentiful, supporting, diluting Nourishment is absolutely necessary to keep up the Spirits, and repair the Loss of the daily wasting Juices, and mend the remaining: Indeed, when the Patients are too heavy and stupid, they should be very frequently prompted to it; for it is even altogether as necessary as Medicine.

We have very seldom any Thing compleatly critical in this Fever; in many Cases only Time itself seems to wear it off. The Urine is scarce ever concocted, but crude, pale and thin thro' the whole Course of the Disorder, and frequently much too profuse; sometimes indeed, after the Exacerbations, or in the Sweats, it is higher coloured, but without Sediment, small in Quantity, and commonly greasy as it were.

It seems to me evident, that too great a Lentor of the lymphatic and most exalted Juices of the Body, is one of the conjunct Causes of slow nervous Fevers; and I conceive, that as the *Serum*, when once coagulated by feverish Heat, never resolves into any Fluid fit for the Uses of the animal *Œconomy*, but turns into an acrimonious *Putrilage*; so the ropy, stagnant Lymph corrupts by Degrees into a putrid *Ichor*, which must be discharged from the Body by its common Outlets, or some artificial Drains. Though the Pores of the Skin, and the salival Ducts, are found in general to be the most advantageous Ways; yet it often partly runs off also by the Intestines and urinary Passages.—Now though these Discharges are many Times very profuse, it is found by Experience, they are not to be too hastily suppressed, without causing a very dangerous Translation of the morbid Matter on the vital Parts: A sudden Check of the Sweats being most commonly attended with convulsive Rigors, vast Uneasiness and Oppression on the *Præcordia, Syncope,* &c;—as *Nausea*, Sickness at Stomach, Colics, and a Delirium are the common Effects of potent Astringents prematurely administered.—Nay the Blisters in this Case are not to be hastily dried up; the more they discharge generally so much the better; and even if they ulcerate somewhat, it is commonly no unfavourable Symptom; for though it may shew the Acrimony of the Humor drained off, it is a Proof that Nature hath Strength enough to expel it:—So that, when the first Blisters begin to heal up, others should be applied to other Parts; for it is not merely from the *Stimulus*, but also from the Drain they make, that they are serviceable.—The large angry Pustules, that often break forth at or after the State of this Fever, and frequently ulcerate and run largely, are a Kind of natural Blisters, which give Vent to the putrid corrosive *Ichor*, and sufficiently indicate one Way of giving Nature Relief.

Upon the whole then, where any of these Discharges are very immoderate, they may be prudently restrained, but not repelled: and therefore cold Air, cold Linnen, cold Liquors, or a cold Regimen, are greatly improper.—And yet to be always labouring by very hot Cordials, volatile alcalious Salts, and very hot Air to raise Sweats, and to continue them is really melting, not mending your Patient. And as to a vast Number, and repeated Eruptions, of the *white and red miliary Pimples,* they not only shew the Quantity of the Disease (as we call it) but many Times also the wrong measures of the Physician. Do we succeed the better for throwing out a vast Number of the Small-pox by a very hot Regimen? And yet the latter bids much fairer for a compleatly critical Discharge than the former.—And I appeal to all experienced Physicians, whether ever they saw large and profuse Sweats of any Service in the Small-pox, or Measles: I am sure I have very many Times found them highly detrimental.

I have been the larger on this Head, as I am fully persuaded, the common Method of treating miliary Fevers by very hot, sweating Medicines, and Regimen hath been the Bane of Thousands.—In a Word, whether in miliary Fevers, or the slow nervous without Eruptions, the sole End of Medicine should be to assist Nature in her Operations, and support her under them; but in such Manner as may comport with the general Laws of the animal Œconomy; promoting by Art, where the Discharges are deficient by Nature, or restraining when profuse and inordinate; taking Care at the same Time never to pervert, in any particular Disease, any particular *Crisis*, which by just Observation, and long Experience, hath been found regular, constant and salutary, but always to favour it.—Thus, to give an Instance in the Fever now treated of; when a *Diarrhœa* happens too profuse, it may be restrained by a gentle cordial Opiate, as *Theriaca Andromachi*, or the like, which by quieting the Irritation, and promoting the cuticular Discharge, moderate the Flux; for gentle, easy breathing Sweats are always found advantageous.—To stop it at once, by very strong Astringents, is to pervert Nature's Endeavours, as they tend to prevent both Stool and Sweat.—But whoever will be more fully informed of the Method of treating the slow nervous Fevers, may consult a late judicious Treatise of Sir *Richard Manningham* on the *Febricula*, &c.

CHAP. VIII.

Of putrid, malignant, petechial Fevers.

LET us next take a View of the putrid, malignant, or pestilential, petechial Fevers, and then proceed to offer some few Directions as to the Method of Cure.

The highly putrid, malignant, and even petechial Fevers many Times arise from mere antecedent Acrimony of the Blood, agitated by the supervening Fever, yet generally the pestilential and petechial have their Origin from Contagion; and may therefore affect persons of all Constitutions, which will of Course produce a great Diversity in the Symptoms.—For, as the received Contagion acts nearly in the same Manner as Acrimony, it will have very different Effects, when it invades a strong vigorous Constitution, and a rich fizy Blood, from what it will, when it attacks a weak, lax Habit with a poor thin Blood, and a too loose *Crasis* of its Globules; and from one and the other, when it falls in with a very acrimonious Mass of Humors.

In general however these Fevers attack with much more Violence than the slow nervous, the *Rigors*, if any, are greater (sometimes they are very great) the Heats much sharper and permanent, yet at first sudden, transient and remittent: The Pulse more tense or hard, but commonly quick and small, though sometimes slow and seemingly regular for a Time, and then fluttering and unequal.—The Head-ach, Giddiness, *Nausea* and Vomiting are much more considerable, even from the very Begining.—Sometimes a severe fixed Pain is felt in one or both Temples, or over one or both Eyebrows, frequently in the Bottom of the Orbit of the Eyes.—The Eyes always appear very full, heavy, yellowish, and very often a little inflamed. The Countenance seems bloated and more dead-coloured than usual.—Commonly the temporal Arteries throb much, and a *Tinnitus Aurium* is very troublesome: A strong Vibration also of the carotid Arteries comes on frequently, in the Advance of the Fever, tho' the Pulse at the Wrist may be small, nay even slow: This is a certain Sign of an impending Delirium, and generally proceeds from some considerable Obstructions in the Brain.

The Prostration of Spirits, Weakness and Faintness are very

often surprisingly great and sudden, tho' no inordinate Evacuation happens; and this too sometimes when the Pulse seems tolerably strong.—The Respiration is most commonly laborious, and interrupted with a Kind of Sighing, or Sobbing, and the Breath is hot and offensive.

Few or none of these Fevers are without a Sort of *Lumbago* or Pain in the Back and Loins; always an universal Weariness, or Soreness is felt, and often much Pain in the Limbs.—Sometimes a great Heat, Load and Pain affect the Pit of the Stomach, with perpetual Vomiting of *porraceous*, or *black Choler*, and a most troublesome *Singultus*; the Matter discharged is frequently of a very nauseous Smell.

The Tongue, tho' only white at the Begining, grows daily more dark and dry; sometimes of a shining livid Colour, with a Kind of dark Bubble at the Top; sometimes exceeding black; and so continues for many Days together; nor is the *Tinge* to be got off many Times for several Days, even after a favourable Crisis: At the Height of the Disease it generally becomes vastly dry, stiff and black, or of a dark Pomegranate Colour.—Hence the Speech is very inarticulate, and scarce intelligible.

The Thirst, in the Augment of the Fever, is commonly very great, sometimes unquenchable; and yet no Kind of Drink pleases, but all seems bitter and mawkish: At other Times however, one is amazed to find no Thirst complained of, tho' the Mouth and Tongue are exceedingly foul and dry this is always a dangerous Symptom, and ends in a Phrenzy, or Coma.—The Lips, and Teeth, especially near the State, are furred up with a very black tenacious *Sordes.*

At the Onset of the Fever the Urine is often crude, pale and vapid, but grows much higher coloured in the Advance, and frequently resembles a strong *Lixivium*, or *citrine Urine*, *tinged* with a very small Quantity of *Blood*; it is without the least Sediment, or even Cloud, and so continues for many Days together: by Degrees it grows darker, like dead, strong, high-coloured Beer, and smells very rank and offensive.—I have frequently seen the Urine, in petechial Fevers, almost black, and very fœtid; particularly that of one Mr. *Shirley*, a Sea-Surgeon, was almost quite black, with a Sediment as dark as Soot: He had Abundance of very black Spots, *Vibices*, bloody Dysentery, and comatose Phrenzy, and died about the thirteenth Day.

The Stools, especially near the State, or in the Decline of the Fever, are of the most Part intolerably stinking, green, livid, or black, frequently with severe Gripes and Blood.—When they are more yellow, or brown, the less Danger; but the highest, when they run off insensibly of whatever Colour. It is likewise a very bad Symptom, when the Belly continues hard, swoln, and tense after profuse Stools; for this is generally the consequence of an Inflammation, or Mortification of the Intestines.—A gentle Diarrhœa is often very beneficial, and sometimes seems the only Way Nature takes to carry off the morbific Matter.

When black, livid, dun, or greenish Spots appear, no one doubts of the Malignity; the more florid however the Spots are, the less is to be feared; it is a good Sign, when the black, or violet *Petechiæ* become of a brighter Colour.—The large black, or livid Spots are almost always attended with profuse Hæmorrhages.—The small dusky brown *Spots*, like *Freckles*, are not much less dangerous than the livid and black; tho' Fluxes of Blood do but seldom accompany them: Excessively profuse, cold, clammy Sweats are often concomitant, by which also they sometimes vanish, tho' without any Advantage to the Patient.—The Eruption of the *Petechiæ* is uncertain, sometimes they appear the fourth or fifth Day, sometimes not till the eleventh, or even later.—The *Vibices*, or large livid, or dark greenish Marks, seldom appear till very near the fatal Period.—We frequently meet with an Efflorescence also, like the Measles, in malignant Fevers, but of a more dull and lurid Hue, in which the Skin, especially on the Breast, appears as it were marbled, or variegated: this in general is an ill Symptom, and I have often seen it attended with very fatal Consequences.

Sometimes about the eleventh or fourteenth Day, on the coming on of profuse Sweats, the *Petechiæ* disappear, and vast Quantities of small *white, miliary Pustules*, break out: I have seldom seen this of very considerable Advantage; but, if an itching, smarting, *red Rash*, it commonly greatly relieves the Sick; and so do the large, fretting; watery Bladders, which many Times rise up on the Back, Breast, Shoulders, *&c.* A *scabby Eruption* likewise, about the Lips and Nose, is certainly one of the salutary Symptoms; and the more hot and angry, it is so much the better.—But of much more uncertain and dangerous Event are the brown dark-coloured *Aphthæ*; nor are those that are exceeding white, and thick like *Lard*, of a very promising Aspect.—They are soon succeeded by great Difficulty of swallowing, Pain and Ulceration of the *Fauces, Œsophagus*, &c. and with an incessant *Singultus*: The whole *primæ Viæ* become at last affected, a bloody Dysentery comes on, followed by a Sphacelation of the Intestines; as is evident from the black, sanious bloody Stools, horribly fœtid, and extreamly infectious.

Vibices, or large black and bluish Marks resembling Bruises, are frequently seen towards the Close of the Fever; and, when attended with Lividity and Coldness of the Extremities, are certain Tokens of approaching Death: I have seen the Blackness reach almost to the very Elbows, and the Hands dead-cold for a Day or two before the Death of the Patient.—A remarkable Instance of this Kind I met with some few Years since in one Mrs. *Hopkins*, to whom I was called the seventh Day of her Illness. She was stupid and somewhat delirious, perpetually sighing, as if under the Extremity of Grief, and complaining of infinite Load and Oppression at her Heart. She had a very quick, small, trembling, unequal Pulse, and a short, catching, laborious Breathing; she had no Manner of Sleep for a long Time, and yet lay very stupid; she had no great Heat tho' insatiably thirsty; the Tongue was not very dry but blackish, her Throat was somewhat sore, and she swallowed with Difficulty: Her Eyes were staring, fixed and inflamed.—The eighth Day she had exeeding profuse Sweats, her Tongue grew quite black, or rather livid, and extreamly dry: In the Evening the *Catamenia* broke forth and became very immoderate, (she was a Nurse, and this was the first Time they appeared since her Delivery) the Sweats continued, and were of a very ill Smell. The ninth they discovered *Vibices*, or large black Spots on several Parts of her Body, one in particular on the Top of her Nose, and another on the Bridge of it, which turned quite black, as did a large Blotch on each Cheek nearly of the Breadth of a Crown-piece.—The tenth the *Catamenia* ceased, she fell into a violent Purging, her Belly swelled exceedingly. Her Nails and Hands grew very black, and as cold as Marble: The Urine and Stool ran off involuntarily, she lay altogether insensible till the eleventh Day, and then died.—An intolerable Stench arose from her at least forty Hours before her Death, tho' kept clean with all possible Care.

I am very sensible, the Word *malignant*, as applied to Fevers, hath of late Years fallen into very great Disrepute, and probably it hath been often made Use of to cover Ignorance, or magnify a Cure.—But there is really a Foundation in Nature for such an Appellation at least for some Word, that may distinguish such a

Disease, as I have been now describing, from a common inflammatory Fever; indeed the very Term *inflammatory Fever* supposes there are other Kinds of Fevers.—It is perhaps indifferent whether you call them putrid, malignant, or pestilential;—when *Petechiæ* appear, every one calls them spotted or petechial,—and, if from Contagion, contagious.—I will contend with nobody about Words, but it is necessary we should have some to communicate our Ideas, and, where they are well defined, no one hath great Reason to quarrel with them.

I have the utmost Honour for the Memory of the great *Sydenham;* and yet, I must say, had he not treated all Fevers as merely inflammatory, even the Plague itself, his Practice had been more universally just and imitable, as being extreamly well adapted to those, that depend on an inflammatory Lentor.—But surely it is not always to be followed, even in the Small-pox, which in general he hath admirably well described and most judiciously treated.—Without all Doubt there are Fevers, that require something more than the Lancet, small Beer and a Purge. Is the low nervous Fever to be treated so? Are some Kinds of Small-pox and petechial Fevers, the miliary, *&c.* to be so managed? I appeal to all experienced and rational Practitioners.—But Honour to whom Honour is due: He justly opposed and exploded the hot, sweating, fiery Regimen, which was then commonly used in all Kinds of Fevers, and introduced proper Evacuations, and the cooling diluting temperate Regimen: A Method most certainly right in all Kinds of inflammatory and ardent Fevers.—Yet mere Evacuations, and cold watery Diluters will not indifferently suit all Sorts of Constitutions and Fevers.—But Opposition is commonly carried too far, and a favourite Notion may sometimes lead one to *extinguish almost the vital Flame,* and *another* to fire the Fabric, lest the *deleterious Miasmata* should make a Lodgment in it.

If a Fever be an Effort of Nature to throw off some offending, or morbid Matter, as most certainly it is, surely it will not be always proper to check it.—The hot Fit of a Tertian, by attenuating the Lentor of the Humors, and removing the Obstructions in the Extremities of the capillary Arteries, terminates the Paroxysm.—Improper Bleeding and Purging often protract it greatly, and make it both anomalous and dangerous.—When the Contagion of the Small-pox is received into the Blood, it produces a Fever, which in a mild Kind of them soon ends in a compleat Eruption, and thence ceases; the Fever, or the Effort of Nature, having expelled the morbific Matter.—But many Times from profuse Evacuations, immoderate Fear, Sinking of the Spirits, and improper Management, she hath not sufficient Vigor to expel the Disease by a proper *Crisis*; but the Pustules are pale, wan, sessile, and remain crude and without any regular Maturation.—And this often is the Case in other eruptive Fevers, even the Plague itself.

The Reason we have to bleed therefore, in the Begining of such Fevers, is to prevent the Fever from running too high, and producing Inflammations of the Brain, Lungs, or other vital Parts; which a great Fulness of rich, dense Blood, violently moved and heated, is very apt to bring on.—In Truth Bleeding in a contagious Disease, as arising merely from Contagion, seems not indicated; because the Contagion is intimately mixed with the Humors, and, by drawing off a small Part of the Blood, you very little lessen the whole Contagion, which will have its Effect, more or less, whether you bleed, or bleed not.—And we find, by the Experiment of Inoculation, that the least Quantity of the variolous Matter, introduced into the Blood, will produce the Small-pox: And we see the same in other Cases, whether the Bite of a Viper, or mad Dog; in the latter of which, by the bye, a small Wound is generally found worse than a large lacerated one; because this gives a more free Vent again to the Poison.

When you have intimately mixed any Ferment with a Liquor to be fermented, you cannot destroy the Fermentation by drawing off Part of the Liquor; for every Part of the Liquor, when in fermentation, is a Ferment; so Contagion received into the Blood operates on, and in every Part of it.—By cooling indeed, adding Acids, *&c.* you may moderate the Fermentation; and, when it is too violent, you may prevent the Splitting of the Vessel (if too full and close shut) by giving proper Vent: So in contagious Fevers, by drawing off Blood you may lessen its Quantity, and prevent it from overdistending, inflaming and rending the Vessels, and lessen the Heat: which might otherwise very greatly augment the Force of the Contagion, and turn the whole Mass of Humors into a mere inflammatory Glew.—But if, to carry on the *Simile,* you cool the fermenting Liquor too much, and prematurely suppress the Fermentation, you render the whole vapid and ropy, and it never purifies itself by a proper *Despumation,* or becomes a good, vinous Liquor.—Thus when Contagion is received, if you weaken the Powers of Nature too much by Bleeding, *&c.* and hinder her Operations in *despumating* (as *Sydenham* calls it) the morbid Humors; you concentrate the

Disease, which turns the whole Mass of Blood into a putrid *Ichor,* or *Sanies.*—However, as Bleeding may lessen the Fewel, tho' it doth not extinguish the contagious Fire, it is highly proper where there is a Redundance of Blood.—But yet the Infection will have its Effect; and I have seen as numerous, and as bad a Kind of Small-pox, after profuse Bleeding, as ever I did when it had been omitted.—It is certain moreover that the Plague, which stands first in the List of contagious Fevers, will very seldom bear Bleeding, to any Degree at least, as appears from the very best Authorities.

But let us finish this Chapter with a few Words on the curative Intentions, proper in the Fevers, which it particularly treats of.—And here first let me note, that tho' malignant and pestilential Fevers, at the very Onset, greatly sink the Spirits, and cause surprising and sudden Weakness, especially when from Contagion; yet Bleeding to some Degree is most commonly requisite, (nay necessary in the Strong and Plethoric) not only to lessen the *Moles movenda*, and give a freer Play to the oscillating Vessels; but also to prevent any inflammatory Obstructions, which may form in the very Begining, and likewise to moderate the Friction and Heat, which are often very considerable for the first Days of the Disorder, and which more and more exalt the Salts and Sulphurs of the Blood, encrease the Acrimony, and putrescent State of the Humors, and greatly favour the Action of the morbific Matter.—This therefore, when indicated, should be done as early as possible.—A quick tense Pulse, sharp Heat, great Difficulty of Breathing, Palpitation of the Heart, and violent Pain on the Head and Back evidently demand it.—But it should be duly observed, that tho' a *Rigor* precede the Heat, and the Oppression on the *Præcordia* be very considerable; yet much less Blood should be taken off than in a true Peripneumony, which oftentimes makes its Attack much in the same Manner: But the sudden Weakness and great Dejection of Spirits, the Trembling of the Hands, the Paleness and Crudity of the Urine, together with the Absence of a Cough, and Heat of the Breath, which attend true peripneumonic Fevers, distinguish the one from the other. Besides this Affair is less liable to be mistaken, when putrid, pestilential, or petechial Fevers are common, and the Constitution of the Air disposeth to them.—Whatever be the Case, the Blood drawn will soon shew the Difference, which, in malignant Fevers, is of a much more loose Contexture and softer Consistence (tho' it may appear very florid) than that of pleuritics, or peripneumonics; which tho' it may, at the first Bleeding, appear very bright, and without a tough white Pellicle on it, especially if it trickles down the Arm, and doth not run off in a full Stream, yet when cold it will form into a very firm and dense *Crassamentum.*—When you find it quite otherwise, be cautious, in all Cases, and not too prodigal of the vital Fluid.

Now, though it may be necessary to bleed the Strong and Robust at the very Begining of contagious Fevers, yet we should have a very careful Regard to the Nature of the Fever, as arising from Contagion, which seems to affect not only the *Blood,* but primarily also the *animal Spirits:* I think the sudden Damp, weakness, Tremblings, and great Dejection of Spirits, at the very Attack, evidently shew it.—In some Plagues Persons have been struck dead as with a Blast of Lightning, without any precedent Fever, or even Indisposition.—It is impossible to account for the immediate Operation of the Bite of a Rattle-snake, which kills often in less than a Minute or two, on any other Supposition; nor for the Surprisingly sudden Effect of some Smells, on some Persons, which almost instantaneously throw the whole Frame of Nature into the utmost Confusion, and even Convulsion.—The now well-known Effects of the Stroke of *electric Effluvia* not only seem to confirm this Notion, but also shew the analogous Manner in which it is done.—Whoever would see more of this, may consult the illustrious Dr. *Mead*'s *Introduction to the third Edition of his Essay on Poisons.*

But the Nerves and animal Spirits, being affected by the contagious *Miasmata,* do not sufficiently and regularly actuate the muscular Fibres and Vessels; whence arises great Debility, and too weak a Vibration of the vascular System; and hence the Blood in some Places runs into grumous Concretions, and in others is quite dissolved.—The Heart and its Auricles are found vastly distended with grumous Blood in those that die of the Plague, the Blood recoiling upon the Heart, which hath not sufficient Power to protrude it; but yet the Blood in the other Vessels appears vastly thin and dissolved, insomuch that it frequently runs off *qua data porta: Timoni** and others observe that it is exceedingly difficult to stanch it at the Orifices made by Bleeding and Cupping.—This I have likewise many Times observed in common petechial and pestilential Fevers.

From the peculiar Disposition of the nervous Filaments, and that of the most subtle and exalted Part of the animal Fluids, which

* *See Philosoph. Transact.* No. 364.

so greatly differs in different Persons, arises that astonishing Diversity of Affections even from the very same Cause.—The smell of an Herb, Flower, Musk, that refreshes thousands, makes some particular People faint.—The Stroke of *electric Effluvia* affects different Persons in a very different Manner, at least in very different Degrees; probably not only from the different *Crasis* of the animal Spirits, but also from the different Tension, Strength, *&c.* of the nervous *Fibrillæ:* As musical Strings, of different Length and Tension, will be very differently affected by the same Note.—It may perhaps, in Part, be owing to the peculiar Disposition of the Nerves and animal Spirits, that some are very readily infected by the Plague, Small-pox, *&c.* and some never, although Multitudes suffer around them.

But be this as it will, the Contagion certainly weakens the Force of the Solids, and tends to dissolve the Blood; so that, when we have a Suspicion that a Fever arises from Contagion, we should proceed with Caution in letting Blood, even though the Symptoms may run pretty high at the Begining, and seem to demand the Taking off a pretty-large Quantity.—In malignant Pleuro-peripneumonies and Peripneumonies I have too often seen, and been sorry for very untoward Mistakes in this Matter, particularly in the Years 1740, 1741, and 1745:—And therefore, though the first Bleeding may be very proper, the subsequent may not be so, nay pernicious.—The first Blood frequently appears florid, what is drawn twentyfour Hours after is commonly livid, black, and too thin, a third Quantity livid, dissolved, and sanious.—This is frequently the Case in malignant petechial Fevers: I have sometimes observed the *Crasis* of the Blood so broken as to deposit a black Powder, like Soot, at the Bottom, the superior Part being either a livid Gore, or a Kind of dark green, and exceedingly soft Jelly.—Besides, the Pulse, in these Cases, sinks oftentimes surprisingly after a second Bleeding, nay sometimes after the first: And this I have more than once noted to my great Concern and Astonishment, and that even where I thought I had sufficient Indications from the Pulse, *&c.* to draw Blood a second Time.—So necessary is it therefore to have a due Regard to the peculiar Nature of an epidemic Fever.

Scarce any infectious Fever makes an Attack on any Person, without bringing on a Sickness at Stomach and Vomiting. As the morbific *Effluvia* are swallowed with the *Saliva, &c.* may they not, in Part at least, be washed off and rejected, by co-operating with Nature, in promoting the Vomiting?—By which also any bilious, acrid, putrid *Colluvies,* that may lie in the Stomach, is carried off; which otherwise, by growing more and more corrupt, would produce a Variety of ill Symptoms, and greatly encrease the original Disease.—Besides, Nature many Times strives in vain to discharge by Vomit without the Assistance of Art, and yet as violently, as when a proper *Emetic,* and a *proper Wash,* are made Use of: Nay drinking something to promote the Vomiting makes it both much easier, and much more effectual, and by carrying off the irritating Matter tends greatly to stop the Vomiting. But then I would have this done always by very gentle Means, such as Infusion, or Decoction of *Ipecacoanha, Oxymel scilliticum,* with a slight infusion of Chamomile Flowers, or the like.—The Method of Vomiting by mere warm Water I do not approve of, as you are oftentimes obliged to swill down immense Quantities, before you can raise the Vomiting, which sometimes overloads the Stomach to such a Degree, that its Force is not sufficient for the Weight laid on it, and cannot reject it; so that the more you drink, the less capable it is of doing its Office: and thus, being over-distended, it becomes quite inactive, whence dreadful Effects may follow.—In all Cases therefore, if no Vomiting follows after having drank a Pint or two, solicit a Discharge with your Finger, or a Feather, and by all Means beware of that Deluge of Drink, which is too often very preposterously given.—I think, by the Way, the Observation, that the Stomach is utterly inactive, and cannot reject any Thing when over-distended, just as the urinary Bladder when overful cannot render any Urine, shews that *Vomiting* is not solely from the Action of the *Diaphragm* and *abdominal Muscles,* as Mons. *Chirac* and others suppose; for their utmost Efforts many Times produce no Manner of Effect on an overful Stomach or Bladder:—In the latter, we are frequently obliged to have Recourse to the *Catheter.*

If the Vomiting continues, after the Stomach is washed out, give a little *Theriaca Andromachi* out of an appropriate stomachic Mixture, as Salt of Wormwood, Juice of Lemons, Mint-water, *&c.* and apply an aromatic Fotus, or rather a Cataplasm of *Species aromaticæ* with *Theriaca,* which most Times succeeds when every Thing else fails.

Not only the Stomach, but the whole intestinal Canal, should be unloaded in the Begining of these Fevers; but I am sure Reason and Experience shew the Necessity of doing it by very gentle Methods; Clysters of Milk, Sugar and Salt, Laxatives of Manna, Cream of Tartar, *Sal cathartic. Glauberi,* Tamarinds and Rhubarb, are what I would chiefly, if not only, advise. I have too often seen the extream ill Effects of acrid and stronger Purgatives.—* *Hoffman* cautions even against *Senna*. The above soft, easy Emetics and *Eccoprotics*, have this further Advantage, that they may be repeated, and given from Time to Time, as the putrid bilious *Colluvies* drains into the first Passages.—By such Means I never fear to puke, or promote a Stool or two, when indicated, at any Time of the Fever, by a nauseous bitter Taste in the Mouth, Sickness at Stomach, *nidorose* and fœtid *Eructations;* or by too great Costiveness, tumid Abdomen, *Borborygmi*, griping Pains, *&c.*

Tho' *Hippocrates* † advises in general against purging off the crude Humors, in the Begining of Diseases, before they are concocted; yet he allows we may purge in the Begining, when there is a *Turgescence* of the Humors, and they make an Effort to be discharged: thus a *Cholera Morbus* is an Effort of Nature to throw off a superabundant acrid Bile.—When putrid, malignant autumnal Fevers arise from a Redundance of putrescent *adust Choler*, as the Ancients called it, in the Region of the Liver, Stomach, *&c.* which is very often the Case after hot Summers have greatly encreased and exalted the Bile, animal Salts and Oils; we should certainly begin with such gentle Emetics, and Cathartics, as I have mentioned.

Unquestionably the bilious Principle is too greatly predominant in all putrid, malignant, and petechial Fevers.—The Gall-bladder and biliary Ducts are always found full of black or green Bile in those, that die of pestilential Diseases, and so is the Stomach, *Duodenum, &c.* ||—Now if this putrid Bile is not carried off, it grows more and more corrupt, and causes vast Anxiety, Sickness at Stomach, Pain, *&c.* and being reabsorbed into the Blood, creates infinite Evils, greatly irritates the *Genus nervosum*, destroys the *Crasis* of the Blood, and turns the *Lymph* into a corrosive *Ichor*.—Where therefore there are Signs of its being redundant, it should be forthwith discharg'd by Vomit, or Stool, as Nature points out.—I have many Times, with the greatest Pleasure, in these putrid Fevers, seen an amazing Change for the better immediately succeed a Fit of Vomiting, and a Stool or two; where an inexpressible Anxiety, Load on the *Præcordia*, perpetual Sickness, *Eructation* and *Singultus* had preceded. The extream Foulness of the Tongue, Sickness

* *De Febribus petechial, veris. Tom.* IV.

† *Aphor.* z. Sect. I. & Lib. *de Humoribus.*

|| *Traité de la Peste, &c. Paris* 1744, 4to.

and Load at Stomach, with a loathsome bitter Taste, and horrible offensive stinking Breath and Eructations, shew the Condition of the Stomach; and the abominably fœtid, black, bilious Stools the Necessity and Advantage of that Discharge.—Surely if a Poison of any Kind was lodged in the Stomach, or Bowels, we should not hesitate about the Necessity of carrying it off as soon as possible; and truly putrid Bile is little less pernicious than an actual Poison. Commonly about the State of these Fevers, or between the seventh and fourteenth Day, Nature of her own Accord endeavours to relieve herself from the putrid bilious *Colluvies* by Vomit, or loose Stools more frequently; and her regular Operations should always be favoured by Art: and accordingly I generally give a gentle Laxative the eighth or ninth Day, unless I find some Eruption appearing, or a kindly Sweat forbid it.—Till this Time, I seldom use any Kind of Purgative except a little Manna, Cream of Tartar, or the like, at the very Begining, (especially when I have Reason to think the Disease arises more from Contagion than a putrid *Saburra*) ordering however an emollient, laxative Clyster every second or third Day, as there may be Occasion.—This Laxative I repeat from Time to Time as Symptoms indicate, and during the Operation carefully support my Patient with proper cordial Diet, Drink and Medicine. By these Means, I not only prevent the Congestion, and encreasing Corruption, of this putrid bilious Matter in the first Passages, but also its *Reabsorption* into the Blood; and likewise solicit a further Discharge of the morbid Humors into the intestinal Canal, and thence out of the Body. This gentle Method of purging about this Time, in these Fevers, I have for many Years found of very great Advantage; but I protest against the *aloetic, scammoniate Coloquintida* Purgers; which in such a putrid, dissolved, acrimonious State of the Blood are Poisons, not Medicines: and whoever uses them in such a Case, should have the Guts of his Brain purged, if he hath any there.—Nature indeed, without such powerful Stimulants, too frequently over-acts her Part, and runs into a profuse Diarrhoea, a Dysentery, soon fatal if not restrained;—but this most commonly happens from suffering the corrupt bilious Matter to lodge, and putrefy too long a Time, in the Bowels; and the best Way to prevent it is to dislodge it, at proper Seasons, and due Intervals.—When we are threatened with such an immoderate Discharge, we must have Recourse to proper astringent Alexipharmacs, *Theriaca Andromachi, Confect. Fracastor.* Tincture of Roses, red Wine mulled up with Cinnamon, *&c.* but above all, if the Case be very urgent, to an astringent Clyster of *Confect. Fracast.* or *Theriaca Andromachi,* with a small Quantity of Decoction of Tormentil, red Roses, or Japon Earth.—But no small Degree of Prudence is necessary in the Use of it; for it is always of dangerous Consequence to suppress a critical Diarrhoea prematurely; and I think it should never be done without premising a small Dose or two of Rhubarb.—Before I conclude this Paragraph, I cannot but take Notice, that tho' I have very often seen a Diarrhœa critical and salutary at the State, or Decline of these Fevers, I generally find it prejudicial at the very Begining; especially if very thin, serous and profuse.—Nothing more certainly shews a Diarrhœa to be useful, than when a gentle breathing Sweat, or warm Moisture of the Skin, accompanies it.

Tho' Nature very frequently affects to discharge the morbific Matter, in putrid malignant Fevers, by Vomit and Stool; yet her more constant and grand Effort is through the Pores of the Skin.—I solemnly assert, I never saw one of these Fevers compleatly judged, or carried off, till more or less of a Sweat issued.—If it proves moderate, warm, and equally diffused over the whole Body, such as we call a breathing Sweat; if it comes on about the State of the Disease, and the Pulse grows more open, soft and calm a little before, and during its Continuance, it is always salutary:—But if very profuse, cold, clammy, or partial, about the Head and Breast only, we have much more Reason to fear than to hope from it.—If profuse Sweats break forth at the Begining, they are generally pernicious; especially if a *Rigor* supervenes.

But, as these Sweats are always most favourable, when they are more the Work of Nature than Art; they should never be too soon, or too forcibly driven out by violent hot Medicines, Regimen, *&c;* it is sufficient to promote and support them, by plentiful subacid Diluents, and gentle cordial Diaphoretics; such as may dilute and wash off the Salts, contemperate the Acrimony, and prevent the further Encrease of the *Putrescence,* and Dissolution of the Blood, and preserve and strengthen the Tone of the Solids.

But, as Persons of very different Constitutions, both as to their Soilds and Fluids, may be attacked by contagious Diseases, very different Methods of Cure will be necessary in their respective Cases: Those of strong Fibres, and a rich dense Blood, do not require such warm Medicines as are necessary to support the Feeble and Phlegmatic. It should be observed in general however, that as the Blood and Humors in pestilential and petechial Fevers tend to Dissolution, Stagnation and Putrefaction; such Methods as will preserve the *contractile* Force of the Vessels, and prevent the Advance of Putrefaction, are necessary: The vegetable, and even properly prepared mineral, Acids are highly serviceable in the latter Intention; and the subastringent Alexipharmacs are very useful in the former.—But I am very certain, that the Use of volatile, alcalious Salts and Spirits is very hurtful; as they without all Doubt augment the putrescent State of the Humors, and act as so many *Spurrers* on to swifter Destruction:—A very large Use of them, without the Aid of Contagion, being found to bring on a Corruption and Dissolution of the Blood, and such Kind of Fevers, even in the most healthy.—Perhaps the pestilential *Miasmata* themselves are only highly volatilized and subtilized animal Salts:—The Generation of pestilential Fevers, by the putrid Exhalations of dead Bodies, after Battles, Sieges, *&c.* seems to shew this.

What I have said of volatile alcalious Salts, leads me to a Reflexion on the promiscuous Use of Blisters in these Fevers; which by some are deemed the only *Anchor of Hope* in such dangerous Cases: But I think they are many Times too hastily and improperly applied, especially in the Begining, when the Fever runs high, and doth not demand a further *Stimulant;* for the Action of the *Cantharides* is not merely on the Skin, but affects the whole nervous and vascular System: Now when the Irritations and Vibrations are already too great, as frequently happens in the Begining of such Fevers, they are very injudiciously applied. Besides, the Salts of these *Flies* operate much in the same Manner as the volatile alcali Salts, and certainly tend to promote the Dissolution, and consequently Putrefaction of the Blood.—It is true indeed, Nature may sometimes want a *Spur,* nay often doth so, particularly towards the Decline of these Fevers; when the Solids grow torpid, the Circulation languid, the Spirits *effœte,* and the Sick comatose: Here Blisters must be applied, and are of exceeding great Use, at whatever Time of the Fever such a Train of Symptoms comes on.—But, in the above Circumstances, I have very many Times seen very pernicious Effects attend their too early Application; as obstinate *Pervigilium, Delirium,* Suppression of Urine, *Tremors, Subsultus,* &c. I would therefore advise the younger Practitioners, before they deal largely in these *wholesome Severities,* to consult *Baglivi de usu & abusu Vesicantium;* and they will understand him much the better, if they previously read his Treatise *de Fibrâ Motrice, & Bellini de Stimulis.*—Let me further add, that where several Blisters are laid on in any acute Case, the Patient should drink freely of Whey,

Emulsion, or some other subacid and demulcent Liquor; otherwise he may suffer almost as much from the Remedy as from the Disease.

It may be expected I should mention *Camphire* as the grand *Corrector* of the Acrimony of *Cantharides;* and in this View I Frequently use it, well knowing that nothing more effectually blunts the *Spicula* of Salts than this exceeding *fine, volatile, vegetable Sulphur;* even those of mercurial Preparations are greatly softened by it.—But I think, in these putrid pestilential Fevers, it answers a much more important End by promoting a *Diaphoresis,* or easy Sweat,which is universally allowed in such Cases of the highest Service: But nothing more certainly doth this than Camphire, with this further Advantage, that it by no Means heats so much as volatile alcalious Salts, and ardent Spirits.—Besides, its anodyne demulcent Quality makes it vastly serviceable, in quieting the *Erethism,* and bringing on Composure of Spirits and easy Sleep, when Opiates fail, nay augment the Tumult and Hurry.—Indeed, when joined with an Opiate, it is the most certain Sudorific in Nature; and the *Elixir asthmaticum,* or *paregoricum,* is not only in this Respect, but in many others, a most noble Medicine. But whenever Opiates are given in these Fevers, it should be only in small Quantities at a Dose, which may be repeated, as indicated; *Theriaca Andromachi, Mithridate, Diascordium, & Elixir Paregoricum* are without all Doubt much the best. *Camphire* however hath this Fault, that it is very disagreeable to the Stomach, but when dissolved in (or rather intimately mixed with) *hot Vinegar,* after the Manner of the *Julep. è Camphorâ,* it sits much easier, and is a Medicine excellently well adapted to putrid malignant Fevers, and even the Plague itself: For both Camphire and Vinegar are highly recommended, by almost all Physicians, in pestilential Diseases. The *French Physicians* made great Use of both, with Success, in the late *Plague of Marseilles,* &c. and *Heinisius* * had a Statue erected to his Memory, for the Service he did in the Plague at *Verona* by a Medicine, the *Basis* of which was *Camphire.*

Now, as we are obliged to give Acids and Subastringents, in putrid malignant and petechial Fevers, to preserve the *Crasis* of the Blood, and the *Tone* of the Vessels, and prevent the further *Putrescence* of the Humors: Diaphoretics (the chief of which is Camphire) should be joined with them, to keep up a free Perspiration, or gentle Sweat, which the former are apt to retard: This is quite conformable

* *Vid. Etmuller. de Pesle Tom.* i. *p.* 263. *Edit. Francofurt,* 1688. *Fol.*

to the Practice of the Ancients, who mixed Astringents with Alexipharmacs, in the Composition of their *Antidota*, as may be seen in *Theriaca Andromachi, Mithridate*, &c.—I am persuaded they are better for it.—These have stood the Test of Ages, and are unquestionably excellent Medicines (when well used) tho' there may be several Things in them trifling both as to Quantity and Quality.—I very well know *Alum* and *Nutmeg* may be given with Advantage, in other Fevers, besides Intermittents; especially when a little *Camphire* and *Saffron* are joined with them.

Here I beg Leave to insert the following *Preparation of the Bark*, which I have used for many Years with success, not only in intermittent and slow nervous Fevers, but also in the putrid, pestilential, and petechial, especially in the Decline; and that too many Times though the Remissions have been very obscure, and yet with a very good Effect.—But, if the patient is costive, or hath a tense and tumid Abdomen, I always premise a Dose of Rhubarb, Manna, or the like.

℞ *Cort. Peruv. opt. pulv.* ℥ii. *Flaved. Aurant. Hispal.* ℥*iss. Rad. Serpent. Virgin.* ʒiii. *Croc. Anglic.* ℈iv. *Coccinel.* ℈ii. *Sp. Vini Gallici* ℥xx. *f. Infusio clausa per dies aliquot (tres saltem quatuorve) deinde coletur.*

Of this I give from ʒi to ℥ss every fourth, sixth, or eighth Hour, with ten, fifteen, or twenty Drops of *Elixir Vitrioli* out of any appropriate Draught, or diluted Wine.—This I order to be kept, in these Parts, as an officinal Medicine; and as a very useful one I recommend it to the Trial of others.—I very well know it will sometimes succeed in Intermittents, when the Bark in Substance, or Decoction, will not easily sit with the Patients: And this is often an Advantage of medicines given in a liquid Form, which in a solid one proved disagreeable; and therefore where it can be conveniently and effectually done, it should be complied with.—The above Composition tends to strengthen the Solids, to prevent the further Dissolution and Corruption of the Blood, and in the Event to restore its *Crasis*:—And this it doth without shutting up the Pores of the Skin too much, which the Bark in Substance too frequently doth.—For it should be noted, that tho' very profuse Sweats in these (and all other Fevers I think) are prejudicial; yet gentle, easy, moderate Sweats are always to be encouraged, particularly at the State, and in the Decline, by proper plentiful Diluents, liquid Aliment, *&c.*—Indeed, as these Fevers very often run out to a great Length of Time, supporting Drinks and Diet are necessary, without which the

Patients certainly sink under them.—In this View, and in those abovementioned, I cannot but recommend a generous *red Wine*, as a most noble, natural subastringent Cordial, and perhaps Art can scarce supply a better.—Of this I am confident, that sometimes at the State, and more frequently in the Decline, of putrid malignant Fevers, it is of the highest Service; especially when acidulated with Juice of Sevil Orange, or Lemon.—It may be also impregnated with some Aromatics, as Cinnamon, Sevil Orange Rind, red Roses, or the like, as may be indicated; and a few Drops of *Elixir Vitrioli* may be added.—I will not say in the Rant of *Asclepiades*,* *Utilitatem vini æquari vix deorum potentiâ*; but it is undoubtedly of admirable Use not only in common Life, but as a Medicine.—*Rhenish* and *French* white Wines, diluted, make a most salutary Drink in several Kinds of Fevers, and generous *Cyder* is little inferior to either.—And, as I said above, sound, old, red Wine is a fine subastringent cordial Julep.—The *Asiatics*, and other Nations, where pestilential Disorders are much more rife than with us, lay more Stress on the Juice of Lemons in these Fevers than on the most celebrated Alexipharmac. It is not as to these only, but in many other Things, that we seek from Art, what all-bountiful Nature most readily, and as effectually, offers us, had we Diligence and Sagacity enough to observe, and make Use of them.—And I cannot but here take Notice, that I think the *dietetic* Part of Medicine is not so much studied as it deserves.—I am sure it is the more natural Way of Cure, tho' less pompous indeed than alexipharmac Bolus, febrifuge Draught and cordial Julep.

As I think the following Dissertations will more fully illustrate and confirm the preceding Doctrine, I shall here subjoin them.

* *Plinii Histor. natural. ex Edit. Harduin. Paris.* 1723, *Folio, Tom. II. p.* 301.

AN ESSAY ON THE SMALL-POX.

THE *different Effects* of the *same Disease*, on *different Constitutions of the Solids and Fluids*, is in no Case more evident than in the *Small-pox*.—For, *first*, when the variolous Contagion attacks a Person of strong tense Fibres, and a rich dense Blood, commonly a smart inflammatory Fever ensues; in which sometimes the Lungs, sometimes the Brain, the Throat and other Parts are greatly inflamed, and on Bleeding you have a very thick inflammatory Blood; and you are many Times obliged to bleed repeatedly, unless you will suffer your Patient to be carried off by a raving Phrenzy, or choaked by a peripneumonic Inflammation.—Here the Pulse is rapid, full, tense; Breathing hot, short, and laborious; the Heat very sharp and the Urine high-coloured; the Thirst great; the Tongue dry and foul; the Pain of the Head, Back, Loins, and Limbs, exceedingly acute.—Under such Symptoms I would bleed in a Pestilence, or indeed any other Disorder whatsoever, or else the utmost Danger will arise from the inflammatory *Diathesis* of the Blood, abstracted from the Contagion.

But I can by no Means approve of the promiscuous Use of Bleeding, so commonly practised in all Attacks of the Small-pox.—For, *2dly*, that Disease many Times comes on with the usual Symptoms of a slow nervous Fever, and the Sick are frequently a long Time *drooping*, as the Vulgar call it; the Fever low, the Spirits sunk, the Pulse weak, quick and fluttering, the Countenance pale and fallen, the Urine crude and thin, no great Thirst, no great Heat, a continued Giddiness and Heaviness, of the Head with Tremblings, a perpetual *Nausea* and Puking, universal Uneasiness, Weakness, Weariness, *&c.* I have several Times known Symptoms of this Kind continue for seven or eight Days together, and at last end in the Small-pox; which almost always proved of a very bad Sort, pale, crude, pitted and *sessile*, never rising well, or maturating kindly, but continuing flat and flaccid, or running together in large watery Blisters, full of thin, undigested *Ichor*, and so remaining to the very last; whilst in the Face, from a deadly pale cadaverous Hue, they turned to a ghastly black, and very adhesive Crust, if the Patient survived long enough, and even then generally proved fatal.

3dly, Sometimes the Small-pox are attended with a Fever of the malignant or petechial Kind, in which the *Crasis* of the Blood becomes quite dissolved, black and livid Spots appear, Hæmorrhages ensue, and the Pustules turn black, gangrenous, and often bloody soon after the Eruption, and that too sometimes when the Pox are very few and distinct.—Here then we find three different Kinds of Fevers produced by one Species of Contagion, and we are obliged in the Method of Cure to have a Regard to the particular Fever, as well as to the peculiar Nature of the contagious Disease.

By this we see how absurd the general Notion of either the *hot*, or *cold Regimen* is in all Kinds of the Small-pox indifferently.—Sometimes *Sydenham's* Method may be proper, sometimes *Morton's*.—In a Word, the particular Case requires a particular Method, and the attending Physician is to shew his Judgment in adapting it rightly.

Tho' the Contagion of the Small-pox produces the same specific Disease, yet the Degrees of that Disease are vastly different.—Even the very same Contagion, in the same House, Family, or Village, frequently produces very different Kinds of Pox; some exceeding mild and distinct, some highly malignant and dangerous.—We see innumerable Instances where the first seized shall have a very favourable Kind, the subsequent a confluent, malign and fatal: This is every Day's Experience; and yet amidst all this, and from the very worse Sort, intermediate Instances happen of the most benign.—So that it is quite Demonstration, that the Constitutions of the particular Patients greatly diversify the succeeding Disease:—And it is so in all Cases; for even a common Scratch in one rankles and proves a stubborn Ulcer, in another a large lacerated Wound heals up with little or no Difficulty.—A common *Phlegmon* in one easily resolves, or suppurates kindly, in another it proves gangrenous, scirrhous or cancerous.

The Contagion of the Small-pox doth not always bring on a Fever, at least to any considerable Degree, though it may the Small-pox; for many Children, and even grown Persons, have had them in the natural Way, in so mild a Manner, that they have had no perceptible Fever, nor scarce ailed any Thing previous to, or during the Course of them.—The variolous *Pus* oftentimes infects the Skin of those that have had them already, producing a great Number of Pustules, altogether similar to those of the Small-pox, of the same Duration and Manner in Maturation, but without any Fever.—This is very common among those that attend and handle Persons ill of that Distemper, especially those who have fine and tender Skins.—Here the Contagion affects the cutaneous Glands, *&c.* only, and not the Blood, which had such an Alteration made in it by the former Small-pox, as not to be susceptive of it ever after.—There are some peculiar Constitutions, that will never receive this Disease; for several Persons never have the Small-pox, though frequently conversing with, and even attending People in them. I knew an *old Nurse* and *one Apothecary*, who for many Years attended Persons (and a great Number too) in the Small-pox, and yet never had them. Nay many, that have industriously endeavoured to catch the Infection, by frequenting the Chambers of the Sick, have done it without Effect;—and yet some of these very Persons, some Months or Years after, have been seized with the Small-pox.—The variolous *Pus*, in *Inoculation*, will not infect every one; and it is well known the *Pus*, even from the same Person, produces very different Numbers of Small-pox in different Persons, and very different Degrees of Fever.—Upon the whole then it is evident, that the previous State of the Body, and Disposition of the Humors, greatly contribute to determine the Quantity and Quality of the Small-pox.—Not but that the contagious *Miasmata* may be of a much more virulent and active Nature at one Time than another, or during one Constitution of the Air than another: and indeed we actually find that it is so.—But even this may be very much owing to that peculiar State of the Air, inducing such or such Qualities into the Solids and Fluids, which render them liable to such and such peculiar Fevers:—For we find one Constitution of the Atmosphere disposeth to inflammatory Fevers, another to the slow nervous, remittents, intermittents, *&c*; and a third to the putrid, malignant, or petechial.—Now where the Contagion coincides, and co-operates with such or such a Constitution, it will be productive of such or such a Kind of Small-pox, or rather of such or such a Kind of Fever with the Small-pox.—For surely we many Times observe a very untoward Fever to accompany the Small-pox, where very few, and very distinct, though of an ill Kind.—Indeed, I think, I have frequently observed the common epidemic Fever manifestly concurring with the Small-pox, and that the variolous Contagion only diversified the Disease; or rather the epidemic Fever was coincident with the Small-pox on the same Subject.—This was the Case very often in 1740, 1741, and 1745; when a violent epidemic Fever, of the pestilential Kind, raged *here*, chiefly among the *Sailors, Soldiers*, and *Prisoners* (especially in the last of those Years) who had commonly the most evident Symptoms of the malignant Fever with the Small-pox, which therefore proved exceeding fatal among them; whereas many Persons in the *Neighbourhood*, that had no Communication with the *Hospitals*, and were otherwise tolerably healthy, had a very favourable Kind.—And probably this malignant Fever was Chiefly owing to the high scorbutic ill Habit of Body, Manner of Life, Confinement, *&c.* to which the above Set of People were subject:—Though I think the Fever*, in 1740, was from another Original.

It should seem then, could we preserve, or produce, a certain peculiar Disposition of the Blood and Humors, we might elude the Force of the Infection: And this indeed is talked of by some, but I think upon a very slight Foundation.—Some particular Preparations of the *Bark* and *Mercurials*, by Way of Antidote, have been thought successful, and I have known some Instances that inclined me to think so; but I am far from being satisfied so far as to advise, or depend on them.

In Truth, in different Constitutions, the very same Medicine shall have very different Effects, and it would be Madness to give the *Bark* and cordial Corroborants to one of very strong rigid Fibres, and a very dense viscid Blood, by Way of *Prophylactic*, or *Preparative;* though they might be of much Service in a weak lax State of Vessels, and a poor watery Blood.—Would Mercurials be proper in a too loosely cohering dissolving State of the Blood?—Verily some bad Effects have been sometimes noted on the Use of them, particularly *Petechiæ*, Hæmorrhages, and profuse *Diarrhœa's* in the ensuing Pox, though I am sensible, in other Circumstances, they may be very useful.—In Sum then, whatever can be done rationally in this Way, must be with a View to mend what is faulty, or supply what is defective, in the Constitution; so as either to fortify it against the Attack of the Disease, or to prepare it the better to cope with it, when it actually seizes.—Perhaps these few Hints may not be altogether

* *Vid. hujus historiam, Obs. nostr. de Aere, &c. Vol. II. mense Junio* 1740.

unworthy the Consideration of those especially, who have the Preparation and Management of Persons to be inoculated.

I am persuaded, if Persons, regularly prepared, were to receive the *variolous Contagion* in a natural Way, far the greater Part would have them in a mild Manner; for undoubtedly a very bad Sort of Small-pox many Times arise from an Over-fulness of Blood, Acrimony of Humors, or great Loads of foul Matter in the first Passages; and very frequently Errors are committed in Diet, Exercise, *&c.* after the Infection is first taken, which often prove of fatal Consequence in the Event.—From these, those that are inoculated are, and should be guarded, and hence the great Success of that Operation.—Not but that the mild Kind, from whence the *variolous Pus* is taken, and the very small Quantity of infectious Matter received by *Insition*, in Part also contribute to the Mildness of the Disease.—This perhaps is the whole of *Inoculation*, if you take in likewise this Consideration, that it is practised chiefly on the young, fearless and most healthy.—Innumerable Instances however have now sufficiently evinced the great Success and Advantage of this Method; and, granting all that Prejudice and Party have said against it, the Danger in the natural Way is at least ten to one, of what it is in this.

A particular Regard then must be had to the Constitution of the Patient, and the Constitution of the Air, if we would practice with Reason and Success in the Small-pox, and indeed in all other epidemic Disorders.

For, *first*, the robust and vigorous Constitutions have more viscid and dense Humors, and much more of the red, globular, compact Blood; and of Course are liable to a higher Fever and greater Inflammation than Persons of lax Fibres, and a poor watery Blood; and for this Reason can better bear, in all Cases, Evacuations, especially by Bleeding.

In the former then it is prudent, on the Attack of the Small-pox, to draw off some Blood, and, if Symptoms run high, to repeat it. A full, tense, throbbing Pulse, great Heat, a difficult and hot Respiration, high Colour of the Face, Redness of Eyes, Phrenzy, *&c.* particularly demand it: An acute Pain of the Head, Inflammation of the Eyes, and Throbbing of the carotid and temporal Arteries, denote an Inflammation of the Brain, or its *Meninges*, which you can never be too earnest and early in endeavouring to remove.—After having drawn a proper Quantity of Blood from the Arm, Bleeding in the Foot hath generally an admirable good Effect.

Bleeding in such Cases doth not retard the Eruption, at least not beyond its due Time.—Where the Blood and Spirits are under a vast Agitation, and the Circulation excessively rapid, Nature is so much embarrassed, as to be unable to make a regular Expulsion of the morbific Matter, much less to *concoct* it, or even to perform the common natural Secretions:—In common ardent and inflammatory Fevers you are many Times obliged to bleed once and again, before you can procure the least Sweat.—Besides, some Degree of *Coction* is necessary in all critical Eruptions, at least in such as prove salutary; and therefore you have generally more or less of a Sediment in the Urine just before, or at, the Eruption, and the Fever subsides.—Where all is in a Hurry, and the Pox are pushed out too soon, frequently even within thirty Hours, the Fever continues, and the Event is almost always fatal.—Nor will Bleeding, under the above Circumstances, weaken the Powers of Nature; but, by calming the over-violent Motion of the vital Fluid, and causing a more regular Secretion of the animal Spirits, it will relieve, nay support her in her Work.

Bleeding in the Foot is known to make a very powerful Revulsion from the Head and Breast, Parts we should endeavour to guard, as much as possible, against the Violence of this Disease.—And, to this End, I would recommend also Bathing the Feet and Legs in warm Water, or Milk and Water, for a few Minutes, two or three Times a Day, before, and at the Eruption; and would likewise have *Cataplasms of Milk and Bread, boiled Turnips*, or the like, applied to the Feet.—This Practice I have for many Years used with Success, and particularly recommended in a short Account, of an anomalous Small-pox, that raged *here* in 1724 and 1725*—This draws the Blood in greater Quantities to the lower Parts, and of Course relieves the Head and Breast; and, as it brings down more Blood, it brings down also more of the variolous Matter to those Parts, and, what is more, facilitates its Eruption on them; which lessens the Quantity, that might otherwise break out about the Head, *&c*: At the same Time the relaxing Quality of the tepid Bath tends to calm the Impetuosity of the Blood, and in some Measure also dilutes it. It is certain, where this Method is used, a vast many Pox break out on the Legs and Feet, and sometimes on the Application of the Cataplasms very severe Pains affect them.—It is the Number of Pustules about the Head, Throat and Breast, that are so justly to

* *Philosoph. Transact.* No. 390.

be feared: A common *Erysipelas* of the Face and Head is vastly more dangerous than on the inferior Limbs.—The Head therefore should never be kept too hot, but should be shaved antecedent to the Eruption, especially where there is much Hair; this not only keeps the Head much cooler and less liable to be over-run with Pustules, but likewise prevents many troublesome Accidents in the Course of the Disease.

If, notwithstanding the Fever continues to run high, the Eruption doth not regularly advance; I would not only advise Bathing the Legs and Feet, but the Arms and Hands, nay and even the Trunk of the Body also.—This I have had Occasion to practise more than once in some Children, who, from being used to the *cold Bath* for ricketty Disorders, had their Skin rendered more dense and hard than natural, which probably retarded the Eruption beyond the due Season. In one of these (now a strong lusty Gentleman) the Pox did not appear till the sixth Day, tho' he had a very smart Fever from the Begining; and then, on bathing him up to the Breast in warm Milk and Water, the Pox came out forthwith, very kindly, though pretty numerous.—Bathing the Body in this Manner not only tends to relieve the Head and Breast, but it also draws out the morbific Matter, and promotes its Eruption on the external Habit, by which the internal and more vital Parts are less liable to the Ravage of the Disease: It is too often found that the *variolous Pustules on the Lungs, Viscera of the Abdomen,* &c. produce mortal Effects.—This is not altogether a new Method: for *Rhazes** advises the Patient to be kept in a kind of *Balneum Vaporis,* to facilitate the Eruption.

Many Times the Strong and Plethoric fall into a vast Dejection of Spirits, and a general Debility, attended with a heavy oppressed Pulse, at the very Seizure with the Small-pox; which makes the less experienced Practitioner very diffident as to Bleeding, tho' here equally necessary, and nothing sooner relieves them, especially when this, in great Part, arises from Fear and Dread of the Disease: which is very often the Case with adult Persons, who by the bye can best bear Bleeding, unless very old. For not only the Contagion itself perhaps primarily affects the animal Spirits, but the very Fear and Concern also so disturb and weaken the Powers of Nature, that the Heart and contractile Vessels exert much less Force on the contained Fluids; whence the regular Secretions and Excretions are considerably diminished, particularly those important ones, the

* *Vid. Rhaz. de Variolis & Morbillis Cap.* vi. *ex Edit. Mead.*

nervous Fluid, and Perspiration: so that hence the *Moles movenda* is encreased, and the *Vis motrix* lessened.—Drawing off Part therefore of the encreased Blood, under such Circumstances, is in Event equivalent to an Encrease of the moving Force.—Besides, when Part of the viscid Humors is drawn off, the remaining are more easily attenuated, and rendered more fit to give off the actuating Principles, or animal Spirits, in due Quantity.—Some Blood therefore, in such Cases, should be drawn as early as possible, but not in too large Quantities at once.—It is certainly better to repeat the Bleeding, if necessary, at least to stop the Orifice now and then; for by this Means you avoid the Fainting, which otherwise frequently happens, unless the Patient is bled in a recumbent, or lying Posture.

But further, where immoderate Fear and Dejection of Spirits concur with the Disease, there is really oftentimes a Necessity of giving something of a cordial Nature, even at the very Begining, and that too sometimes even not sparingly. Now when the superabundant Quantity of the Blood is drawn off, these invigorating Medicines may be used with greater Safety and Advantage; and I have many Times seen exceeding good Effects from them, where the Pustules, thro' excessive Fear, and Oppression of Spirits of the Patients, lay buried in the Skin, as it were, and made no considerable Advance for two or three Days together.—I am no great Advocate for the *hot Regimen*, especially at the Begining of the Small-pox; but I know this must be done in such Cases, and Blisters must be applied to rouse the sluggish Oscillations of the Vessels, or the Patient certainly sinks under the Malady.—Yet in general, I am not fond of Blistering very early in the Small-pox, unless there is great Reason to fear that the Tongue, *Fauces*, and narine Passages, are otherwise like to be greatly infested with them: When the Disease attacks with a Rawness, Soreness, or great Heat of the Mouth and Throat, and a considerable sharp *Rheum*, or Stoppage in the Nostrils with frequent Sneezing, and a tickling Cough; this is to be expected, unless prevented by timely Blistering, which I have often found very successful.—A great Sneezing, and sharp *Rheum* from the Mouth and Nostrils, shew that the *Membrana Schneideriana*, the common Lining to all these Passages, is greatly affected, and that a Revulsion from it is indicated; for even a few Pustules in the Throat and Nostrils are of vastly worse consequence than an hundred Times the Number on the external Habit: Great Pain and Difficulty of breathing and swallowing are the certain Effects, especially towards the Close of the Disease; which frequently quite choak the Sick, unless you are exceeding diligent with your Gargles, Syringing, *&c.* Sometimes I have known such a violent Defluxion on these Parts, as to cause a very profuse Salivation even at the very Begining; which hath kept the Patient constantly awake, excoriated the Tongue, Lips and Throat, and brought on such excessive Pain as utterly to deprive them of Sleep, and make Swallowing any Drink, Aliment, *&c.* almost intolerable: Here early Blistering in the Neck, behind the Ears, *&c.* is indispensably necessary.

But secondly, when Persons of weak lax Fibres, and a poor thin Blood, or those, who have undergone lately great Evacuations, are attacked with the Small-pox, withhold your Lancet as you tender the Life of your Patients.—These generally have a sunk pale Countenance, a weak, quick, trembling Pulse, very great Dejection of Spirits, with a pale crude wheyish or limpid Urine, alternate Chills and Heats, little Thirst, and no great Pain, but a perpetual Heaviness and Sickness at Stomach, Giddiness, *&c.* Here, I pronounce it, *Sack and Saffron* are not improper, with some easy, cordial, nervous Medicines, Sack, Whey, Wine and Water, or the like.—But all this may be done without large Doses of volatile alcalious Salts, and Spirits, Snake-Root, Brandy, strong Wine, *&c.*—And yet I have seen pretty large Quantities of Wine given in some low depressed Cases, with very great Advantage: Blisters also may be here applied, and stimulating Cataplasms to the Feet; Bathing seems not so proper.

There is one Thing in a peculiar Manner, that greatly promotes the variolous Eruption in these low slow Cases, where the Pustules do not break forth in a regular Manner, at the usual Season, but lie buried in the Skin with little or no Protuberance, and less Colour; and that is *Vomiting* by a *gentle Emetic.*—Nature almost always makes this Effort spontaneously in this Disease, and I think we should follow the *Indication*; for it not only in Part throws off the morbific Matter, which primarily affected the Stomach, but also the heavy putrid bilious *Colluvies*, that may have been collected in it, the Liver, Gall-Bladder, *&c.*—It is very notorious that the Action of Vomiting forces off through the Skin, Perspiration, Sweat, Pustules.—I know it is objected, that Vomiting drives up too much Blood to the Brain; and therefore is improper in the Begining of the Small-pox: and I think so too, if done antecedent to Bleeding in plethoric Constitutions; nay I have known very terrible Accidents ensue, where thus injudiciously managed.—But let it be considered, that, without the Solicitation of Art, Nature is always at it, and makes almost perpetual, tho' many Times vain, Endeavours to discharge the Stomach: Now it is certain, that by co-operating with her Motions, and assisting her Effort with a proper *Wash*, we greatly help her Attempt, and the Vomiting even ceases much the sooner; and it is observable, that on the compleat Eruption the Vomiting goes quite off, but even that is by this Means very much promoted. —I would have the Cataplasms to the Feet immediately succeed the Emetic, for Reasons that are very obvious.

The Emetic hath commonly the further good Effect of producing a Stool or two, by which the Intestines are unloaded of gross, indurated Excrements, or any putrid bilious Contents; if this doth not happen, an emollient laxative Clyster should be forthwith given: And, in many Cases, a gentle, easy, cool Cathartic of Manna, Cream of Tartar, *Glauber*'s Salt, or Rhubarb is necessary; even if a Diarrhoea is urgent, a Dose or two of Rhubarb should be given.

Different Constitutions of the Air have different Effects on the most healthy, much more on the sick and weak, and of Course on Diseases.—It hath been long observed, that one Constitution of the Atmosphere promotes, another retards the Progress of epidemic disorders, particularly of the Small-pox; which at one Time begin in the remotest Corner of a Town or City, and soon ravage the whole; at another they are carried into the very Heart of them, and yet presently cease.—The Plague itself is commonly stopped, by a Change of Air from hot and moist to cold and dry.—The very State of the Blood greatly depends on the precedent and present Constitution of the Air, and it hath been proved, that the Contagion hath different Effects on different States of the Blood.—A due Consideration therefore of the present, and preceding Constitution of the Air, is of no small Import in our Method of Cure.

As a continued cold dry Air makes the Fibres strong and very elastic, and the Blood dense and viscid; one may reasonably conclude, that Patients, in such a Constitution, will *cæteris paribus,* more need, and better bear Blood-letting, than in a warm, moist, relaxing State of the Air; and that they will want more of the diluting, emollient *antiphlogistic* Drink, Diet and Medicines: whereas in the latter something more cordial, subastringent and *antiputrescent* will be requisite.

It is certain, in very cold and dry Weather, as also when very hot and dry, Persons in the Small-pox spit vastly less than in the opposite Constitutions of the Air; so that in a very dry Atmosphere all proper Means should be used to dilute the Humors, and promote

Salivation, so necessary and salutary in this Disease:—This however in some Seasons, and some Persons, is vastly too profuse and prejudicial; I think more particularly in coldish, moist, flabby Weather, and in Persons subject to catarrhal Disorders.—I have many Times known the *Salivation* begin so soon, and continue so immoderate, as at length to abrade the common Invelop of the Tongue, Mouth and Fauces, causing most exquisite Pain, preventing Sleep and Swallowing, and keeping the Patients in a perpetual Torture.—And therefore I always dread a *premature Salivation*, especially when profuse and very acrid.

As some Constitutions of the Air hinder a sufficient Salivation, others dispose to too much, and that too acrimonious: An epidemic Catarrh shall at one Time be only a Discharge of a thin, soft, insipid *Mucus*; at another, a profuse acrid *Gleet*, excoriating the Nose, Lips, Fauces, *&c.*—Probably such a Kind of Atmosphere, as disposes, to excessive Salivations, may in Part also be productive of that crude, *crystalline, undigested Pox*, which we too frequently meet with. For a moist, flabby, chill Season not only too much relaxes the *contractile* Vessels, and impregnates the Blood with the cold nitrous Vapors; but withal greatly obstructs Perspiration, whence a sharp, serous *Colluvies* is accumulated; and it is chiefly, in such Seasons, that this Sort of Small-pox is predominant; as the small, warty black Kind, with little or no Salivation, is most commonly observed during a long continued Course of dry North-Easterly Winds, very hot or very cold dry Weather.—Doth not this Observation hint to us the different Regimen necessary in different Seasons?

These *crystalline*, or *lymphatic* Pox never maturate kindly, but the Matter remains crude, and a mere watery *Ichor* to the last, and in many Places they run one into another, and form very large Vesications; which at length breaking and corroding all around them, the Patient is ulcerated all over, and appears like a flead Rabbit.—I have seen some running down under such a Kind of a *Tabes* for twenty or thirty Days together, the sharp Humors ouzing out, and dripping from them continually, till at last they have been *dissolved in a double Sense.*—Very frequently a great Part of this thin crude Matter is re-absorbed into the Blood, and leaves a vast Number of the Pustules flaccid, empty, or *siliquose*, as they call it. This creates terrible Disorders, and plays over the Tragedy again, which generally ends in a fatal *Catastrophe*; convulsive *Rigors*, peripneumonic Fever, Delirium, Dysentery, *Syncope, &c.* are the common Consequences.—However when it goes off by a moderate

Diarrhœa, or a very plentiful Discharge of full-coloured subsiding Urine, the Sick very often recover; but when the Stools are black, bloody, or sanious, they generally indicate a Mortification of the Intestines, especially if the Abdomen is swoln, painful and tense.—And a *Micturition*, or perpetual Urging to Urine, without any considerable Discharge, is a very bad Symptom, unless it arises from Blisters.—If ever large Sweats are useful in the Small-pox, it is in this Kind of them; and I think I have found them several Times greatly advantageous.

In this *crude, ichorose, indigestible Pox* and profuse *Ptyalism*, where the Skin and Pustules are pale, or lurid, the Pulse weak, the Urine thin, watery, crude; the warmer Medicines are necessary: such as *Pulv. Contrayerv. c. Myrrh, Musk, Saffron, Camphire, Theriaca, Mithridate, Confectio cardiaca.* These are of vast Service in raising the Pustules, and digesting the Matter, and may be washed down with Sack-whey, *Decoct. rubicund.* a temperate testaceous Julep, *or a Dish of Coffee* now and then with a little thin Milk in it; which I have known, more than once, drank thro' the whole Course of the Small-pox with no ill Effect, nay with a very good one; as it manifestly quieted the tickling vexatious Cough caused by the sharp thin Rheum.

Here also without Doubt Opiates are strongly indicated, and *Theriaca, Elixir paregoricum,* or *Tinctura Thebaica* should be given with *Diacodium* frequently, but in such Doses as to quiet, not to stupefy the Patient; which indeed is the most safe Method of giving Opiates in all Sorts of Fevers, and ultimately the most effectual; for tho' a large Dose at once may more immediately procure Sleep, yet it is much less refreshing; but, when it doth not, a Delirium is almost always the certain Consequence, or a long continued Stupor.—In all Events great Doses cause very great Relaxation and universal Debility, which nothing but a fresh Dose after some Time, or a warm Cordial will relieve: They are similar in Effect to large Doses of *spirituous Liquors*, which produce temporary Madness, or Stupefaction, ending in general Weakness, Tremors, and the utmost Dejection of Spirits.—Besides, no one can say, what Effect a particular Dose of Opium will have on a particular Person, till he hath tried it: Some have such a peculiar Disposition, that a very small Dose will greatly affect them; whereas others of nearly the same apparent Strength, Constitution, *&c.* will take four times the Quantity with vastly less Effect.—Some bear *Diacodium* that cannot touch *Opium*: So that it is always prudent to begin at least with moderate Opiates, and in small Doses.

Yet notwithstanding this Caution, there are no Medicines whatever that incrassate thin acrid Humors, abate their Irritation and Defluxion, and maturate the Pustules, so effectually as Opiates properly given.—In Truth, when the Pustules are numerous, we can do very little without them, especially towards the State of the Disease, when they become exceeding painful.—And yet even here, when the Salivation is extreamly viscid and difficult, and the Respiration short and laborious; we should be very cautious in using them, and join with them *Gum ammoniac, Oxymel scilliticum,* &c.

Nor must we in this *lymphatic, or crystalline Pox* be sparing of Blisters, which, besides their other good Effects, give a copious Vent to the acrid morbific Humors; and for the same Reason the large Bladders, which the Pustules cause by running together, should be opened with a Lancet.—Letting out the Matter with a golden Needle, as **Avicenna* advises, is more nice than necessary. Do it as you will, a worse *Cicatrix* follows than when committed to Nature: But here the Danger supersedes that Consideration; for a Mortification is sometimes brought on by the corrrosive Matter, and some of it withal is continually re-absorbed into the Blood.

I would also advise some proper Diuretics to be joined with the alexipharmac Medicines, as *Nitre, Sal Succini, Spirit. nitri dulcis,* and the like. For I have many Times observed a plentiful Flow of Urine very happily compensate the Deficiency of other Evacuations: and, if this happens when the Salivation begins to cease, and the Face subsides, it is always salutary; and, as it is so, it should be promoted as much as possible; and the Sick should be frequently prompted to discharge it, which is greatly facilitated by getting them up on their Knees. For, whilst lying in Bed, they have many Times neither Inclination, nor Power, to make it; and yet immediately, on being lifted up, they shall render it in a large Quantity.

Nothing is more common than for the thin, acrid, variolous Matter to take a Turn down the Intestines, and very often in a very violent Manner.—Innumerable Instances have occurred in the Small-pox, where a critical Diarrhœa hath saved the Life of the Patient; Nature even substitutes this Discharge in Children, for the Salivation in Adults.—We should be very Careful therefore never to suppress it too hastily; and even when it is profuse, we should not

* *Avicenna Canon. Medic. Lib.* iv. *Cap. de. Variolis, p.* 66. *ex Edit. Plempii.*

attempt it, till we have premised a Dose or two of Rhubarb; and then indeed proper Astringents, Opiates, *Decoct. rubicund. Decoct. Fracast. Tinct. Ros.* &c. may be used; and, when every Thing else fails, a Clyster with *Diascordium*, or *Theriaca*, will stem the Torrent. But in general we should only moderate it, especially at, or after the State, taking Care however to support the Patient during the Flux with a proper strengthening, subastringent Diet.

I never observed either the *vegetable or the mineral Acids* of any great Service in the crude crystalline Pox, but I have often found them highly useful in the *small, black, confluent Kind, with Petechiæ*; in which the Putrefaction of the Humors in general seems much greater, and the Matter of the Pustules is vastly more fœtid and sanious than in the *crystalline*, the *Ichor* of which many Times hath little or no Stench at all.—Tho' perhaps scarce one in four recovers from this small, black, confluent Kind (and when attended with black Spots, bloody Urine, and other Hæmorrhages, scarce one of a thousand) yet sometimes great Things have been done by mineral Acids, astringent Alexipharmacs, and Preparations of the *Cortex Peruv.* when the *Petechiæ* have been numerous, and the Small-pox very black, small, and confluent, nay, and even attended with some Degree of Hæmorrhage.—I have known some Instances of a Recovery, under these Circumstances, by those Methods; but never met with one, who survived the Disease, that made bloody Urine, unless it was manifestly from *Cantharides.*—But as this Kind of Pox is of very long Duration, and the Patient (if he at length gets over it) continues between Life and Death as it were for many Days together; the above Medicines are not only necessary, but he should be also plentifully supported, in the *last Stadium* especially, with proper *analeptic* and *antiseptic* Drinks and Diet; till at last, like the Serpent, Emblem of recovered Health, he crawls out of the *black Exuviæ* into new Life and Vigor: and truly I have seen some Cases, which seemed more like a Resurrection than a Recovery.

When I recommend the Use of the *Bark*, in some Kinds of the Small-pox, I do it upon sufficient Experience and Authority; whoever is not satisfied with mine, may consult the great Dr. *Mead**, Prof. *Monro*†, and Dr. *Wall*‖ on this Matter.—I commonly begin with the *alexipharmac Tincture of the Bark* above described,

* *De Variolis & Morbillis, p.* 45.

† *Medical Essays, Vol.* v. *p.* 102.

‖ *Philosoph. Transact.* No. 486.

well acidulated with Elixir of Vitriol; and then proceed to the Decoction, or Extract, if necessary.—But let me strongly caution against giving any Thing of this Kind, where the Respiration is difficult, the Body very costive, and the Abdomen hard and tumid, at least till you have removed those Symptoms.—I must add, that the *Tinct. Cort. alexipharm.* is particularly serviceable in the *lymphatic Pox*, and should be given soon after the compleat Eruption, to promote, as much as possible, some Degree of Maturation: It is certain the *Bark* commonly brings on a laudable Digestion in gleety Ulcers.—*Morton** gave the Bark, not only in the *Decline*, but during the *Maturation* of the Pox, if he found any Remission; and that too every third or fourth Hour, to the Quantity of a Drachm; and I know this hath been practised many Years ago with Success by some other eminent Physicians.

The great Difficulty and Danger of this Disease chiefly comes on at the *State*, or *Turn* of the Pox (which happens much sooner in some Kinds than in others, the milder the Pox, always the sooner;) for however easily Matters may have proceeded till this Time, we are now (*viz.* the seventh, ninth, or eleventh Day from the Eruption) very often surprised with a very shocking Change, and terrible Symptoms. The Swelling of the Face sinks at once, the Salivation suddenly ceases, the Pustules grow flaccid, the Interstices pale, lurid, or ash-coloured: a Rigor comes on, a Fever succeeds with great Difficulty of Breathing, Faintness and Sickness; a perpetual Anxiey, Tremors, Subsultus, Delirium, *&c.* soon follow.—Such a Change is to be expected, if the Pustules break out very numerous the first, second, or third Day from the Seizure; if after the compleat Eruption they do not fill well, keep up round and properly pointed, but grow flat, and run abroad, or have a small *Dimple*, or *black Speck* in the Middle; if they are not surrounded with a *florid Base*, and look themselves wan, or darkish coloured:—If the Urine withal hath continued, or grows pale, crude, and thin, and the *carotid* and *temporal Arteries* throb much, no small Danger is impending.—Here then the Physician must in a more especial Manner watch his Patient with the utmost Diligence; for the Affair of Life and Death is now to be transacted in a few Hours:—and, though no absolute Rules can be well laid down in a Disease, that is attended with such a great Variety of Accidents as the Small-pox; yet perhaps the following Hints may not be altogether useless.

* *De Variolis, cap.* ix. p. 250.

1st,—If the Swelling of the Hands doth not regularly succeed the Tumor of the Face, and the Swelling of the Feet that of the Hands, it is justly reckoned an ill Symptom; for this is a regular and critical Translation of the morbid Humors to those Parts, and commonly happens when the Salivation begins to abate, and the Face subsides. Where therefore Circumstances are threatening, I would advise the Application of Epispastics to the *Wrists and Ancles*, a little before we expect the Tumor of the respective Parts should come on; for these not only more certainly draw the Humors there, but also gives them Vent: And I think the Use of emollient *Cataplasms*, or *Fotus*, to the Parts should for some Time precede the Blisters, as they would also tend to solicit these critical Tumors.—*Baglivi** says he ordered Sponges soaked in emollient Decoctions with great Success.—Sometimes indeed Nature, of her own Accord, throws the morbid Matter on the Extremities with such Violence, as to create great Inflammation, Tumor and most exquisite Pain; which nothing will so effectually relieve as emollient Fomentations, by relaxing the Parts, and opening the Pores.

The foregoing method I recommended above twenty Years ago†, and have since practised it in Abundance of Instances with great Advantage.—The premature Recession of critical Tumors is always of very dangerous Consequence, witness even the common Gout: insomuch that we are many Times obliged to fix it by acrid Cataplasms.—In the above Case Blisters not only attract, but discharge, the morbific Matter. I very frequently add *Cantharides to the Cataplasms*; and I find it is now a Practice with some very great Physicians to apply Blisters to the Soles of the Feet, in Cases of Danger.

2dly.—If Heat, Head-ach, Sickness and Load at Stomach, great Restlessness, or Stupor, come on about the sixth or eighth Day from the Eruption, the Body being costive, as most commonly it is; a plain Clyster of Milk, Sugar, and Salt, seldom fails of giving immediate Relief: and this is especially necessary, when the Sick make frequent but vain Efforts to Stool. For the Excrements, baked up by Heat and long Retention, are crowded into the *Colon* and *Rectum*; where pressing on the Bottom of the *Aorta, Iliacs*, and Neck of the Bladder, they hinder the free Descent of the Blood to the lower Parts, whence the Head and Breast are overloaded: Besides, they

* *De Variolis & Morbillis.*

† *Philosoph. Transact.* No. 390.

suppress the Urine, and neither Wind, Stool, nor Water, can be discharged till the indurated Excrements are softened, and the Guts relaxed, lubricated, and irritated to their Office by a proper Clyster.—Indeed I seldom suffer my Patients, particularly young Persons, to grow so exceeding costive: for I generally order an emollient Clyster, if necessary, to be injected every second, third, or fourth Day from the very begining, till I enter on the Use of gentle Purgatives; which keeps the Patients much cooler, and renders the Use of Anodynes much more safe and effectual: For very often they will have little or no Effect, till the Body is unloaded, or bring on a comatose Disposition.

And yet, *3dly,*—Anodynes are almost always proper, nay necessary, in the Small-pox, especially at and towards the Crisis: were it for nothing but to asswage the Pain from the Inflammation of the Skin and Pustules, they would be required; for if one Boil is attended with so much Uneasiness, what will ten thousand occasion? However the Pain and Soreness complained of, is generally a good Symptom:—It is certainly a very bad one, when neither the Skin nor Pustules inflame or grow painful; for it argues a great Deficiency of the *Vis Vitæ*, Want of a due Circulation in the extream Capillaries, and an universal *Torpor.*—Let me further add, that towards the State especially, the Opiates should be given early in the Evening, before the Exacerbation comes on, and in larger Doses; and if Need be, oftener repeated.— *Diacodium* here seldom proves sufficient, unless in Children.—The Dose of the Anodyne particularly should be always encreased the Evening before we expect the Crisis, in order to quiet the Tumult, which generally comes on the ensuing Night; for, as *Hippocrates** observes, the Night before the Crisis, in all Fevers, is most troublesome. When the Patient is very feverish and hot, I find it best to give the Opiate with some *Acid*, or out of a *saline Draught*; but, when low and languid, with *Theriaca*, or some *Alexipharmac.*

4thly,—If at the Approach of the secondary Fever the Pulse beats very quick, hard and strong, the carotid Arteries throb greatly, the Heat grows intense, the Breathing very difficult, and an acute Pain of the Head, or more or less of a Phrenzy comes on; you are to bleed immediately, or in a very short Time the Case will be irrecoverable.—It is observable, that the Blood drawn, under such Circumstances, is extreamly viscid, and as buffy as in the highest

* *Aphorism* 13. *Sect.* ii.

Pleurisy: It is very evident, that it is in a very inflammatory State, from the Ophthalmies, Quinsies, Peripneumonies, Rheumatisms, and external Inflammations, which commonly succeed.

But *5thly*,—If on the contrary the Pulse flags, the Patient faints, the Pustules and the Interstices grow pale, shrivelled and sunk, or livid, the Extremities coldish or clammy; you can scarce give too warm Medicines, Drinks, *&c.* nor apply too many Blisters: I have seen very large Quantities of warm Wine given under such Circumstances with surprising Success.

6thly,— About the Close of the *third Stadium* of the Small-pox, the Salivation commonly abates much, and the Matter very often grows so exceeding thick and glutinous, that it is spit off with the utmost Difficulty, and threatens Suffocation every Minute almost, unless perpetually deterged by proper Gargles, Syringing, *&c.*—I know no *Gargles* better in this Case than *Cyder* and *Honey*, or *Vinegar, Water,* and *Honey*, or *Oxymel scilliticum*, with a little Nitre or crude *Sal ammoniac.* Mustard also may be boiled with Advantage in the Gargles, when a stronger Stimulant is wanting.—The vegetable Acids are much more saponaceous and abstersive than Spirit of Vitriol, though more commonly used.—Many Times all these are ineffectual, and nothing but an actual Vomit will relieve; *Sydenham* vomited in this Case with *Vinum benedictum to* ℥iss.—We have much milder but equally efficacious: nay *Oxymel scilliticum* frequently given many Times succeeds, by gently puking, and easing both Expectoration and Respiration.—Besides it hath the further Advantage of promoting Urine, and Stool, which are very often deficient at this Time of the Disease; but, when the Case is urgent, it should be quickened by a Decoction, or Infusion of *Ipecacoanha.* I have had Honesty and Resolution enough to put this in practice several Times, where this was the *derniere Ressource*, and thereby have sometimes evidently snatched my Patient from the Jaws of Death, though at the Risque of my own Reputation; but truly sometimes also I have lost both.—But I shall ever be of *Celsus's* Opinion, to try a doubtful Remedy rather than none.—It is not very uncommon to find the Tongue and Fauces covered with a vastly thick, adhesive, whitish, or brown *Pellicle*, so that they look as if they had been *parboiled*; and the *Oesophagus* and *Aspera Arteria* are commonly in the same Condition: This neither Vomit, Gargle, nor aught else will remove, and is a very bad Symptom, as it shews there is no Manner of Secretion through the Glands of the Parts.

The great Tenacity of the Mucus of the Mouth, Fauces, *&c.* many Times arises from Want of drinking freely, through the Course of the Distemper.—But this is absolutely necessary to dilute the Blood, support the Salivation, fill the Pustules, wash off the morbid acrid Salts, and supply the Vessels with more wholesome Fluids: The very Aliment in this Disease should be, nay must be, chiefly liquid; as Solids, for the most Part, can be neither relished, nor swallowed.—In the black, confluent Small-pox you must drink, or die:—Thin acidulated Whey, *Decoct. Lusitan.* Gruel, or Water with Rhenish or small French White-wine, Cyder and Water, or the like, are exceeding proper; and if either petechiæ, or Hæmorrhages, appear, Tincture of Roses, or Claret and Water well acidulated.

But, 7*thly*,—When the Incrustation is perfectly formed, and the Salivation abates, we must study to promote some other Evacuations; for nothing now is to be further thrown off on the external Habit, little or nothing now can transpire through the crusty, scaly Skin, which invelopes the Body like a Coat of Mail, or rather, in its Consequences, like the poisonous Shirt of *Hercules*: for it not only vastly hinders Perspiration, but also confines the *Pus* and *Sanies*, which grow every Hour more and more putrid, and, being continually resorbed into the Blood, bring on, feed, and augment the secondary Fever.

If we can keep up the Salivation, and promote a due *Flow* of well concocted Urine, at this Period, Things go on tolerably well; but, very often, they both greatly fail all on a sudden, and the Patient falls into the utmost Danger.—Here all Endeavours should be used to renew these Evacuations; more Blisters should be forthwith laid on, and an emollient laxative Clyster immediately injected: Expectorating Mixtures likewise of *Oxymel scilliticum, Lac ammoniac.* &c. should be frequently used.

Moreover, it is of no small Advantage at this Time of the Disease to shift the Linnen of the Sick, which is now grown exceeding foul, stiff and stinking, and become vastly uneasy to them:—Besides it very much pollutes the Air of the Chamber, and renders it so very unfit for Respiration, that even the most Healthy can scarce bear it; nay it not only hurts the Breathing, but the *Miasmata* of this poisonous *Mephites* are continually passing into the Blood again through the *Vasa inhalantia*, Lungs, *&c.* and further corrupt the Blood. It is surprising to find how greatly the Sick are refreshed on changing the Air of the Room, by prudently opening the Windows and Doors, and removing the stinking Linnen, *&c*:—They have new

Life, as they frequently and properly express it; for fresh Air is the Breath of Life.—It is certainly of the highest ill Consequence to confine such putrid Air, and the Sick in it.—The absurd Method of making a Kind of *Hospital Chamber* in a House, and crowding up two, three, or more Sick in it, is a most dangerous Practice, and I have often known it manifestly fatal:—The Stench, the Groans, the Cries of one disturb and offend the others; it is rare that they sleep all together, but they are too often kept waking so: It is bad Living by such bad Neighbours.—Whatever may be pretended, there is no Manner of Danger in shifting the Sick, provided it be carefully done into very dry warm Linnen; but it is a silly Notion to have the Shirt, or Shift, worn by another Person for twelve or twenty-four Hours before it is put on the sick Person.—Can it not be made fully dry and warm without so doing? Will not the Perspiration, or Sweat, of the most Healthy dirt and damp it?

But of this enough: I return to the Affair of Evacuation, and shall conclude this Head with some Observations on Purging in the secondary Fever of the Small-pox.

When the Salivation proceeds regularly, the Pustules keep up and maturate kindly, the Swellings of the Face, Hands and Feet come on in due Season, and the Patients sleep quietly, and breathe freely; all Things are well, and Nature is most effectually doing her own Work, and should be properly supported in it, but never disturbed.—Here I even abstain from Clysters, though the Patient may have been costive for several Days together, till after the compleat Incrustation; and then they are proper to prepare for the succeeding Purges, which without all Doubt are then necessary.

But it very often, nay almost always, happens in the *coherent* and *confluent* Pox, at, or before, this Period, that more or less of a *secondary Fever* comes on; partly from the Resorption of the Matter of the external and internal Pustules, partly from the suppressed Perspiration, and partly from the putrid *Colluvies* of the intestinal Canal: which cannot but be very considerable, as undoubtedly Part of the morbific Matter, separated by the Glands of the Mouth, Fauces, *&c.* is swallowed, and a great deal more must be secreted by the Glands of the Guts, biliary Ducts, *&c.* into the Intestines: For, as vastly less than usual now passes off through the Skin, a much greater Quantity of Humors must fall on the Bowels; it being a well known Maxim, that the Lessening of one Evacuation is the Encrease of another, and also that there is a peculiar Consent between the Skin and the Guts: To all this likewise is added the purulent Matter of the variolous Pustules, that may happen to be in the Stomach and Intestines.—So that there cannot but be a great Lodgment of very putrid Matter in the first Passages, which grows the more and more virulent, the longer it continues there, and is perpetually passing again into the Blood, through the *absorbing Vessels of the Guts*, and becomes a Fewel to the Fever, which Nature endeavours even this Way, partly at least to throw off.—Should it remain there then, or should it be carried off? The Answer is obvious.—Nature of her own Accord commonly attempts it with the greatest Advantage in the Adults, and almost always in Children, to whom a Diarrhœa is a Kind of *succedaneum* to the Salivation of elder Persons.—Is not this then a sufficient Indication how to relieve her at such a Juncture? And in Truth, what horribly fœtid, putrid, large Stools do we observe in this Distemper, on the Use of a Clyster, and more especially after a Purgative, I mean at the State, or in the Declination? Nay this Mass of Corruption lying long in the guts, and growing daily more putrid, becomes at last so extreamly acrid as to corrode them; at least so greatly irritates them, as to bring on that very Diarrhœa, or Dysentery, which some so vainly fear will arise from a gentle Cathartic.

But further, if Nature, neither by her own Effort, nor the Help of Art, is capable of keeping the morbific Humors from falling on the more vital Parts, but, from an unfortunate Translation of it, is like to sink under its Weight; as upon a sudden Retrocession of the Tumor of the Face and Hands, a premature Suppression of the Salivation, or the like; doth it not seem necessary to carry off the offending Matter by some other Outlet, as particularly by the Guts, which are much more easily and certainly solicited to a Discharge than the Pores of the Skin, the urinary Passages, or the *salivary Ducts?*—Indeed when the Salivation of Course ceases, in my Opinion, it seems proper to promote some other Evacuation in its Room; and if we use a Clyster, or a gentle Purgative, we may readily restrain too great a Discharge by an Opiate.

It hath, and may be objected to this Practice, that it tends to draw the noxious Humors from the external Habit to the Vitals.—But to this I answer, that Purging is more especially pleaded for, when the Incrustation is formed, and the morbid Matter concocted, at least as much as ever it will be (for a due Concoction, or Maturation, is never to be expected in the lymphatic Kind); that it is particularly contended for, when an unfavourable *Metastasis* of the morbid Matter hath already happened, and cannot well and readily be removed by other Means; that this is substituted in the Place of a suppressed critical Evacuation, and that Nature attempts, nay ultimately requires a Discharge this Way; that there is no other Method of dislodging the putrid Colluvies in the Intestines, that feeds the secondary Fever, but this; and that whenever there is a great Quantity of foul corrupt Matter in the first Passages, of what Kind soever, there is a consequent Fever: witness verminious, capulary, bilious Fevers, which cannot be carried off but by purging and vomiting; lastly, that every one allows the absolute Necessity of purging at the Close of the Small-pox; otherwise Boils, indurated Glands, foul Ulcers, carious Bones, rotten Lungs, or a consuming Hectic, certainly succeed.

But when I recommend Purging in the secondary Fever of the Small-pox, I would always advise to begin with the most lenient cool Cathartics: The *drastic, scammoniate, aloetic Purgers* are certainly highly improper till the Fever greatly abates; then indeed some stronger Purgatives (to which I always join some *Calomel*) should be used. The imprudent Use of strong hot Purges at the Begining, the not giving a proper Anodyne after the Purges, and the Want of duly supporting the Sick during the Operation, have, I am persuaded, been frequently attended with ill consequences; but am very sure, that Purging in the secondary Fever, in the Manner I have advised, is of great Service, and I have seen very many Instances of its great Success.

A DISSERTATION ON PLEURISIES *and* PERIPNEUMONIES.

CHAP. I.

Of the Power of the Winds and Seasons in producing these Distempers.

AS Pleurisies and Peripneumonies are, and always have been, so very common, *Hippocrates* hath said much more upon them than on any other of the acute Disease; and his Observations are found most perfectly just, and will be ever highly worthy of a diligent Perusal by all Physicians.—One of them is, that cold north-easterly Winds bring on Disorders of the Breast, Sides and Lungs*; and this hath been found constant and true by all his Successors.—Not but that Pleurisies, and Peripneumonies especially, are frequently observed in other Constitutions of the Air, the latter very often supervening other acute Fevers: Yet still it is certain, these two Diseases are much more frequent, when a cold dry Season, and northerly and easterly Winds, have continued for any considerable Time.

The obvious Effects of dry cold Winds on the human Body are, constringing the whole external Habit, making the Skin more dry and corrugated, shutting up its Pores and lessening Perspiration, at least suffering only the thinner Part of the Humors to fly off. By a dry Cold also the whole System of the Fibres is made more strong, firm, and elastic, and the Action of the Vessels, on the contained

* *Aphorism.* 5. *Sect.* iii.

Fluids, more vigorous and forcible; whence a brisker Circulation, more Heat, Spirit, and Activity; by which the Globules of the Blood are rendered more dense, compact, and numerous, and the whole Mass of Humors disposed to a greater Degree of Tenacity.—It may be added, that as cold and dry Air is almost always very heavy and elastic, by its greater Pressure on the Body, it will co-operate with its cold and dry Qualities, in producing greater Effects.—It is Fact, that, *cæteris paribus*, Blood drawn, in such prevailing constitutions of the Atmosphere, is constantly found more dense and viscid than in long moist warm Seasons;—and that Persons subject to asthmatic Disorders suffer most during the Continuance of north-easterly Winds.

However all these Effects may consist with high Health, and commonly do so; and therefore *Celsus* (though reckoning up the Disorders produced by cold northerly Winds) says* *sanun tamen corpus spissat, & mobilius atque expeditius reddit.*

But alas! such is the frail Estate of mortal Man, that the Transition from high Health to great Disease is most easy and exceeding common: For this high, rich, dense Blood, agitated by strong and vigorous Vessels, is extreamly apt to be wrought up to such a Degree of Viscidity, as makes it unfit to pass the ultimate Ramifications of the Arteries: from which Obstructions, and consequent Inflammations, most easily arise; especially on any Excess in Diet, or Exercise, on obstructed Perspiration, or any sudden Alteration in the Temperature of the Air, which may rarefy the Humors in general much more suddenly, than it can relax many of the particular Vessels.—Whence, by the bye, those Pains in Limbs, formerly broken, in *Cicatrices* of old Wounds, in callous Concretions on the Toes, *&c.* (where the minute Vessels have been rendered more straitened in their Capacities, and more rigid in their Coats) are observed to rage on sudden Changes of Weather into stormy, or wet and warm; which nothing so soon removes as an emollient Fotus, by enlarging and softening the Vessels:—Every old Woman tells you to soak your Corns, when they pain you.—And this Method also is of very great Service in those Pains of the Side, which often remain after Pleurisies or Pleuro-peripneumonies, for Years together, and which are owing to a preternatural Coarctation of the Vessels by the past Disease, and the Adhesion of the Lungs to the Pleura: And which many Times, on great Rarefaction of the Blood, Changes of

* *Lib. II. Cap.* i.

Weather, *&c.* bring on the Disorder afresh, and make the Patient subject to frequent Returns of it for ever after.

It is true indeed, that Persons of a very viscid State of Blood and rigid Fibres are subject to inflammatory Disorders of all Kinds, in all Seasons; but some Constitutions of the Air however are not only more apt to produce this inflammatory Blood than others, but also dispose more to Inflammations of particular Parts. For when very cold Air constringes the external Habit, corrugates the Skin, and shuts up the Pores, more Blood than ordinary is forced on the internal and more vital Parts, particularly on the Lungs; which, by the vast Expanse of their internal Surface (greatly exceeding that of the whole Skin*) are designed by Nature to assist the Skin, in exhaling off the superfluous acrid and vapid Humidity of the Blood; and therefore, where the Pores of the Skin are in any Degree shut up, the Exhalation from the Lungs should compensate the Defect of the cuticular discharge.—And we in Fact find, that, immediately on taking Cold, the Lungs are more or less affected by Cough, a large Discharge of thin *Rheum*, and very often in a much severer Manner.—But when the very cold Air is likewise continually admitted into the Lungs, it also corrugates their internal Membrane, shuts up its excretory Ducts, and so hinders a due Exhalation, and Expiration, if I may so say, of the Surcharge from the retained *Perspirabile.*—It may be added, that the Air, by its great Degree of coldness and Nearness to the Blood in the pulmonary Vesicles and Cellules, is apt to congeal, at least greatly to condense it: There have been many Instances, where extream cold Air hath caused and absolute and sudden Stagnation of the Blood in the Lungs, and killed almost instantaneously. We find often that very cold Winds so affect, and contract even the Skin of the Hands, Arms, and Face, as to make it rough, cracked, and sore; why may we not suppose it hath a similar Effect on the more tender and delicate Membrane of the *Trachea Arteria, Bronchia,* &c? In Truth the Cough, Hoarseness and Soreness, we commonly feel in breathing such a cold Atmosphere, shew that it really hath so. The *Pharynx* and *Larynx* are very often so affected by severe cold Winds, as to suffer violent Inflammations, Tumors, *&c.*

It is easy to conceive then, where a greater Quantity than ordinary of dense sizy Blood is thrown on the Lungs, and where the Vessels of the Lungs themselves are inordinately constringed, and

* *See Dr.* Hale's Vegetable Statics, *p.* 239.

the excretory Ducts and Orifices of the Glands of the Wind-pipe, Bronchia, *&c.* are considerably obstructed; that peripneumonic Inflammations will be very readily generated.

But further, a very viscid Blood, the natural consequence of a long, dry, cold Constitution of the Air, will not only dispose to Inflammations in general, and to peripneumonic Disorders in particular, but also to the pleuritic. For as the Arteries, expanded on membranous Parts, are extreamly small; they are of Course liable to be obstructed by a gross sizy Blood: And hence Rheumatisms are also very common in such Seasons, the membranous Parts of the Muscles being inflamed by a viscid Lentor.—But the *Pleura* is a Membrane very largely extended, and spread over with an infinite Number of very small Arteries, Ramifications of the Intercostals, which, arising nearly at right Angles from the *Aorta*, by that Means receive the more viscid Part of the Blood, as being the lighter (the heavier passing on nearer the *Axis* of the great Artery) and hence are exceeding subject to Obstructions from an inflammatory Lentor: And so are likewise the intercostal Muscles, and *Periosteum* of the Ribs, which receive the Blood, in Part at least, from a like Distribution of the Arteries.

Hence Pleurisies, as well as Peripneumonies, are found exceeding common, or epidemic, in very cold dry Seasons; and in high, cold Situations, much exposed to north-easterly Winds, they are commonly endemic. Indeed pleuritic Disorders, properly so called, are apt to bring on the peripneumonic, and very frequently do so, for Reasons which will be given hereafter.—Hence it comes to pass, that we find many more Pleurisies complicated with peripneumonic Symptoms, than true and exquisite Pleurisies; and this compound Disease the Moderns very properly call a *Pleuro-peripneumony.*

As these two Diseases are so often conjoined, the Ancients, as well as many of the Moderns, have quite confounded them, ascribing the same Symptoms both to one and the other indifferently; but there is a real Difference certainly both as to the Seat and Symptoms of these two Disorders.—Indeed the Ancients, as *Cœlius Aurelianus** informs us, were greatly divided in their Opinion as to the Seat of a Pleurisy, some affirming it to be an Affection, or Passion of the Pleura, properly so called; others of the Lungs and its Membranes: Both which Opinions have had their respective Abettors also

* *Lib. II. Cap.* xvi.

amongst the Moderns.—I flatter myself, the following Remarks will more fully explain their Nature and Method of Cure.

CHAP. II.

Of the Peripneumony and Pleuro-peripneumony.

A Peripneumony, in the largest Sense of the Word, is a Disease so common, either as an original Malady, or consequent to some other, that its Nature should be diligently studied by every Physician; as it is a morbid Affection of one of the principal Organs of Life, is very frequently attended with the utmost Danger, and requires very different Treatment in its different Stages.—Besides there are very different Degrees, I might say Species, of this Disease, which demand a particular Attention, and a Method of Cure peculiarly adapted to each.

For a Peripneumony, arising from a violent Inflammation of the Lungs, by a very sizy dense Blood obstructing very many of the pulmonic and bronchial Arteries, is a quite different Disease, and requires a very different Treatment from an Obstruction of the Lungs by a heavy, viscid, pituitous Matter; as is the Case in what late Writers call a *Peripneumonia notha.*—And this again should be managed in a Method very different from that, which is proper in one depending on a thin, acrid Defluxion on the Lungs. And yet there are some general Symptoms common to them all, particularly a Load at the Breast, a short difficult Breathing, a Cough, and more or less of a Fever: which few obvious Symptoms however give the general Denomination of a Peripneumony, tho' in Nature very different, and to be treated very differently.—For in the *first Case* speedy, large, and repeated Bleeding is absolutely necessary to lessen the Quantity and Force of the too rapid Blood, with the most cooling, relaxing, diluting Diet and Medicines.—In the *second* some Blood indeed may be drawn off, at the very Begining, to prevent the further Impaction of the obstructing Lentor, and make Room for proper inciding diluting Attenuants; but if you are too busy with your Lancet, you weaken the Patient, not the Disease, which requires Attenuants, Detergents, Expectorants, gentle Pukes and proper Purges, with the free Use of Blisters; which I think are quite naught in the former Case, unless towards the Close of the Disease, when they may be sometimes necessary.—The *third Case* may require Bleeding also, to hinder the Advance of the Inflammation; but here the soft, lubricating, demulcent Method, with some proper and frequent Opiates in moderate Doses, are demanded, which in the *second Case* would be utterly deleterious.

Great Regard must be had also to the different Stages, even of the same Kind of Peripneumony, and the different Symptoms that attend it. For tho', at the Begining of a severe Inflammation of the Lungs, large and repeated Bleeding may be indispensably necessary; yet if, after the second or third Bleeding, the Patient begins to spit off freely a well concocted Matter tinged with Blood, you are to restrain further Evacuation that Way; otherwise you weaken your Patient without Necessity, and often entirely suppress the Expectoration to his utter Ruin.—And yet if a considerable Quantity of thin, florid, spumous Blood is spit off, you should draw more Blood, quiet the Cough with cool Opiates, as *Diacodium*, or the like, and give pretty freely of proper *Acids* with soft cooling *Incrassants*: Whereas if it is a thin, gleety; dark-coloured Matter that is expectorated, it is generally a Mark of greater Malignity, and that the Blood is in a putrefying dissolving State, and will by no Means bear a large Emission of Blood.—In short the Disease is quite another Thing, when the Inflammation is forming, from what it is when the obstructing Matter is concocted, or actually suppurated.

But to be more particular.—If a Person just before in full Health, should on violent Exercise, Debauch, or a severe Cold, be seized with a great Shivering, succeeded by burning Heat, very much Oppression and Load at Breast, with a very difficult, quick, hot Respiration, and more or less of a Cough; Blood is to be drawn immediately, in a pretty large Quantity from a large Orifice: The stronger and more plethoric the Patient, the larger the Quantity, yet so as to stop on the Appearance of Faintness, cold Sweat in the Forehead or Face, Yawning, and the like; which may in a great Measure, many Times, be prevented by bleeding the Person in a recumbent Posture.—In general fat corpulent Persons do not bear Bleeding as well as the lean and muscular, as neither having so much of the red globular Part of the Blood, nor their Vessels so elastic.—Besides the Age and Size of the Person are to be considered: It would be absurd to draw as much from a Dwarf as a Giant, tho' both strong in their Kind; the very young and very old are not the properest Subjects for it, tho' both sometimes require it.

Sanctorius observes, that antecedent to Fevers the Body grows more heavy, and of Course more plethoric; and the *Rigors* shew a *Viscosity* in the Blood, that stagnates in the Extremities of the capillary Arteries: (it may be even seen in the Nails, Lips, *&c.* by their growing pale and livid) and this encreasing *Lentor* will of Course lessen Perspiration, and encrease the Quantity of Humors. —Generally the more violent the *Rigor* or *Horror* is at the Attack, the more violent is the succeeding Fever; and this may in some Measure also guide us in drawing off Blood, as we must expect, on a violent and long continued Rigor, a high Fever, and a very viscid State of the Blood.

If the Symptoms are not relieved by the first Bleeding, after eight, ten, or twelve Hours more Blood should be drawn, nay even sooner if they become more aggravated; and this must be repeated, if the Fever, Oppression, Anxiety and Difficulty of breathing encrease, or continue equally severe: especially if the Blood drawn appears very firm and dense, or covered over with a tough yellowish *Coat*, or *Buff*, as it is called; which however very frequently doth not appear till the second or third Bleeding, tho' the Symptoms may indicate a very high Inflammation.—And this very often happens by the Trickling of the Blood down the Arm from a small Orifice, too strait a Bandage, or by the Sliding of the Skin over the Orifice: by any of which the Blood is hindered from spouting forth in a full Stream.

This dense buffy Appearance of the Blood, with a firm strong Pulse, will warrant the drawing off Blood, till the Respiration at least becomes more free and easy.—But if the *Crassamentum, or concrete Mass,* is of a very loose Texture, and not covered with a sizy Coat or Buff, and the Pulse seems to sink, flutter, or grows more weak and small on Bleeding; it is Time to desist, and try other Methods of Relief.—A thin, bluish *Film* on the Blood, with a Kind of soft greenish Jelly immediately underneath, (the *Cruor* itself being livid, loose and soft, with a turbid reddish or green Serum) is a Sign of a very *lax Crasis* of Blood, and *great Acrimony*, which will not bear large Quantities to be drawn off.—Nay even a very florid, thin, loose Blood, that gives off little or no Serum after standing some Time, however, *specious* it may appear to unexperienced Persons, is far from being the *good Blood* they imagine; but generally argues, in this Disease especially, a very considerable Advance to a putrid and very acrid State: For by mixing Spirit of Harts-horn, or Salammoniac with Blood from the most healthy, as it runs off, it always puts on such a florid Appearance, and gives off little or no Serum, how long soever kept, but still remains loose, and as it were half fluid.—It is observable that Spirits of Harts-horn used frequently, and in large Quantities, dissolves the Blood, and brings on profuse Hæmorrhages; which, I think, is an Observation that should be well considered by those, who take so frequently and freely of that Spirit.

A strong, throbbing, quick Pulse in Peripneumonies always indicates further Bleeding, at least till some Degree of Ease in breathing, or a free Expectoration of laudable Matter is obtained.—But it frequently happens that the Pulse, even at the very Begining, seems obscure and oppressed, irregular, sluggish, and sometimes intermitting, the Patient at the same Time complaining of great Weakness and Oppression, which would seem to contraindicate Bleeding; and yet the Load at Breast, Difficulty of breathing, great Anxiety, and Heat felt about the Præcordia, loudly demand it.—This often puzzles the young Practitioner.—But he should consider, that such a sudden Want of Strength, Spirits, and Pulse, doth not arise from Want of Blood, as the Duration of the Disease for a few Hours, or a Day or two, cannot be supposed to have exhausted the vital Liquid to any considerable Degree.—The Truth is, not the Defect, but the too great Quantity of Blood, in such Cases, is the real Cause of these Symptoms.—For the Blood-vessels being overloaded with Humors, and distended beyond the due Tone, cannot act with sufficient Vigor.—The *Æquilibrium* between the Solids and Fluids being not duly kept up, the moving Vessels are unable to protrude the Blood with a due Force; just as too great a Weight on the *Embolus of a Syringe* hinders its free Play. Hence indeed soon follows a Deficiency of Spirits, from Want of a due Circulation of the Blood, and proper Secretion of them; and thence a Tendency to Stagnation, Concretion, and a large Train of direful Symptoms, and even Death itself, unless timely prevented by sufficient Bleeding; which, by diminishing the too great Quantity of Blood, restores the *Æquilibrium* between the Solids and Fluids, and a free Action to the elastic, muscular Canals, which now again exert more Force on the contained Humors, and carry on the Circulation in a more regular and constant Manner: All which tend to attenuate the too thick and viscid Blood, and render it more fit for the Secretion of animal Spirits, which may further invigorate the Action of the Heart and Vessels.—So that in such Cases, *Letting of Blood* is so far from weakening, that it really raises the Powers of Nature; as is always evident on drawing Blood from plethoric Persons, labouring under an oppressed Pulse, as it is properly called, which is found constantly to rise on bleeding.

In some very violent Peripneumonies, where both the Lobes of the Lungs are greatly inflamed and obstructed, an immediate and excessive Weakness comes on, with an inexpressible Anxiety, and Oppression at the Breast, a very small, weak, trembling Pulse, Coldness of the Extremities, with clammy, coldish, partial Sweats, the Eyes staring, fixed, and inflamed, the Face bloated and almost livid; and all this soon followed with Stupor, *Delirium*; and I have seen in some Cases (though few indeed) with a *compleat Paraplegia.*

This is in Truth a very dreadful Case, but doth not arise from Want of Blood, but from Want of a due Circulation and Distribution of it: For there being so many and great Obstructions in the Branches of the pulmonic Artery, the Blood is ponded up in the Lungs, and hindered from passing freely, as it ought, from the right Ventricle of the Heart to the left; so that the Aorta and its Branches do not receive Blood enough to carry on the common Offices of Life, on which soon follows an absolute Stagnation and immediate Death.—Dissections have shewn this to be the Case, the Lungs having been found quite stuffed up with concreted Blood, red, hard, and as it were fleshy, or rather of the Colour and Consistence of Liver, and so heavy, that any Part of them, cut off, sunk in Water*.—If any Thing can be done in this most deplorable Case, it is by early and immediate Bleeding, or it becomes in very few Hours utterly irrecoverable.—I have seen some surprisingly good Effects from Bleeding in both Arms at once, when done in proper Season.

And yet there are some Kinds of Peripneumonies, that will by no Means bear large Bleeding, as hath been noted by Physicians of the best Authority.—And I have observed the same in several epidemic Peripneumonies, particularly in the latter Part of the Year 1745, and the Begining of 1746†; during which we had an epidemic Peripneumony, in which after a second Bleeding (and even sometimes after a single Bleeding) the Pulse and Strength of the Patients sunk to a surprising Degree; and they ran into a Sort of nervous Fever with great Tremors, *Subsultus Tendinum*, profuse Sweats, or an atrabilious Diarrhœa, with a black Tongue, *Coma*, or *Delirium*; though

* *Vid. Hoffman. de Febribus pneumonicis Obs.* i.

† *Vid. Obs. nostr. de Aere & Morb. epidem. Vol. II.*

at the Begining the Pulse seemed to be full and throbbing, and the Pain, Cough, and Oppression so very urgent, as to indicate Bleeding pretty strongly.—Now in these Cases, the Blood was seldom found *buffy* to any considerable Degree, but commonly very florid, but of a very *loose and soft Consistence,* or *very dark-coloured, and coated with a very thin and bluish or greenish Film,* under which was a soft *greenish Jelly,* and a *dark livid Cruor* at the Bottom.—Sometimes indeed the Coat was much thicker and more *tough,* but of a *pale red Colour resembling the Cornelian Stone, or dilute Jelly of red Currants.*—This last Appearance I have frequently noted in real Pleuro-peripneumonies.—Whenever I see such a loose, dissolved Blood, I am very cautious how I advise further Bleeding, especially if I find the Pulse, or the Patient become more languid after it, however, the Oppression, Load, or even Pain, may seem to require it.—It was from Observations of this Kind that *Lancisi,* and *Baglivi* from him, caution against further Bleeding, when no *sizy Coat* appears on the Blood in the Second Bleeding: *In Pleuritide, Peripneumoniâ,* &c. *si in sanguine è venâ sectâ extracto non appareat in superficie crusta alba,—pessimum;—si vero in altera sanguinis missione incipiat apparere, bonum: contra si in secundâ ne quidem apparebit, abstineto statim à sanguinis missione, aliter intersicies ægrotantem**.—And I concur with *Baglivi* in the first Part of the *Prognostic* as well as the last, having always found the very florid Blood, drawn in the Begining of pulmonic Fevers, of very ill *Omen*; for it shews, that either the *Crasis* of the Blood is much broken and dissolved, or that the gross inflammatory Blood sticks in the pulmonary Arteries, and that nothing but the very thinnest and most serous Part can transude and pass into the left Ventricle of the Heart.

I cannot but observe however, that sometimes in Peripneumonies and Pleuro-pneumonies, the first, and even the second Blood shall not appear buffy, and yet the third shall be very fizy, and this particularly if the Blood trickles down the Arm, and doth not come off in a full Stream; but then it is ever to be observed that this Blood, tho' apparently florid, when cold, is very dense and tenacious; whereas in the Case I mentioned above, the Blood, tho' very florid, was of a very loose and soft Contexture, and never formed into a regular firm Crassamentum.—Such a Kind of loose, dissolved, florid Blood was frequently drawn from *Sea-faring Persons* in the

* *Cap. de Pleuritide.*

Begining of the Year 1746*, and was always attended with very ill Symptoms, very often fatal.—Such malignant Peripneumonies indeed very frequently happen to *Sailors* after long Voyages, and to Persons very *scorbutic.*—They grow first of all very short-breathed, listless, and faint on the least Motion, and have transient erratic Chills, Heats, and Pains all over their Body; a Fever succeeds with a vast Load on the *Præcordia*, and a short, importunate, dry Cough, a very quick, small, and much softer Pulse than usual in true inflammatory Peripneumonies, clammy, unequal Sweats, and a perpetual Restlessness and Anxiety; at last they begin to spit a *thin, gleety, bloody, or very dark-coloured Matter*, frequently of a very *offensive Smell*: Moreover these are not uncommonly attended with an Eruption of red, brown, livid, or black *Petechiæ*. The *Urine* is commonly of a blackish dull Hue, or of a *firey lixivial Colour, as if a small Portion of Blood was dissolved in it*: this is rendered in small Quantities, and without any Manner of Sediment; but the former hath sometimes a large livid *Hypostasis*, sometimes nothing but a Matter like coarse Bran irregularly scattered up and down in it.—As these Symptoms are greatly argumentative of a broken Crasis of Blood, and high Acrimony of the Humors; large Bleeding is not likely to be successful, tho' too often imprudently used.

Though the Appearance of a pretty thick sizy Coat on the Blood is in general no ill Symptom in pulmonic Fevers; yet where it is excessively tough, and extreamly yellow, or of a pale lead Colour, it threatens Danger, and shews the inflammatory Lentor is highly wrought up, and vastly difficult to be resolved or attenuated, and that it will scarce admit of any Commixture with any of the Diluents, that are taken in.—This seems apparent from the *odd Shape*, the *Crassamentum* of the Blood often puts on, of a *globular*, or rather a Kind of an *oblate sphæroidal* Figure, after large and frequent Bleeding in violent pleuritic, or peripneumonic Fevers; for then the Cake of Blood is found to swim in a great Quantity of very thin, and sometimes a quite limpid, Serum; its greatly *contracted concave* Surface, or Coat, being almost as tough as Leather, and the whole Mass nearly as hard and firm as a Piece of Flesh.—Now in this Case, as a great Deal of the globular Part of the Blood was drawn off by repeated Bleeding, the Crassamentum is much lessened in its Quantity; but still retains its greatly morbid Viscosity, and its Globules, being vastly dense, attract one the other exceeding

* *Vid. Obs. nostr. de Aere, &c. Vol. II. Mens. Jan. Febr. Martio.*

strongly, as appears by the Figure and Consistence of the Crassamentum: and tho' the Proportion of the Serum may have been greatly augmented, by the Use of Plentiful Diluents; yet it appears from the Tenuity and Limpidness thereof, that they have not been well mixed and united with the globular, and sulphureous or oily Part of the Blood. Nay it is often observed, that thin, watery Diluents are drank in large Quantities, in these severe Fevers, and rendered off by Urine almost as limpid and insipid as Water*, or run off in vastly profuse Sweats; not in the least mixing, in a due Manner, with the Blood, properly so called, nor in the least acting on the Salts and Sulphurs thereof, their exceeding firm Combination eluding the Force of the Diluters. I have repeatedly seen this in Pleuro-peripneumonies, where the Pain hath remained, almost as violent as ever, after the fourth or fifth Bleeding, and the globular Part of the Blood hath been so reduced, as that the Crassamentum hath scarce been a sixth Part of the Volume of the whole Blood, and yet as solid as a Piece of Flesh.—These Cases are generally mortal.

If after the second or third Bleeding, nay if after the first, your Patient begins to spit off freely a yellowish concocted Matter, lightly tinged with Blood, stop there, and particularly if the Breathing becomes more free, as it commonly doth; otherwise you will weaken your Patient to no Purpose, nay to a bad one, and quite suppress the Expectoration, by which Nature is now throwing off the Disease by the most proper *Crisis*, and ready *Outlet*; the obstructing Matter in the Extremities of the bronchial and pulmonic Arteries being so far resolved, concocted, or digested, as to pass off freely into the Cavities of the *Vesiculæ, Bronchia,* &c. and so up, and out of the *Trachea*, by Cough and Expectoration: whence the extream Branches of these Arteries become again passable, and the Circulation thro' the Lungs at last duly restored.

That there is a Passage from the bronchial Arteries, into the Cavities of the Trachea and its Ramifications, is evident; for the *oily Mucus*, which in a natural State lines and lubricates the internal Membrane of the *Aspera Arteria* and its Branches, is separated from the bronchial Arteries.—And it is also certain that Water, Serum, *&c.* pass freely from the pulmonary Arteries into the bronchial, vesicular Cavities; as appears from the Experiments of

* *Hippocrates* observes that making Water, immediately after Drinking, is a dangerous Symptom in Pleurisies and Peripneumonies, *Coac. Prænot. Sect. V. Ed. Lind.*

Ruysch, and the accurate Doctor *Hales.*—Indeed as the bronchial and pulmonic Arteries, in their different Ramifications, join by innumerable *Anastomoses*; even by this Way the pulmonic Arteries may have a Communication with the *Bronchia.*—Now when the obstructing Matter is so duly attenuated and concocted, and the Vessels so far dilated as to give a free passage; it is thrown into the Cavities of the Bronchia, and so out of the Lungs by Expectoration. It seems evident that the lateral, or serous Branches of those Arteries, at their Extremities, are so far dilatable as in some Cases to pass red Globules, and that too freely, into the Cavities of the Bronchia; as is particularly seen in those Spittings of Blood, which are made *per Diapedesin*, as *Galen* and the Ancients called it; For I think it is pretty certain, that some *Hæmoptoe's* do not arise from a Rupture of the Vessels, as no Manner of Pain, Purulence, or the like, precede, succeed or accompany them.

But where these small Vessels of the Lungs are by Nature or Art made easily dilatable, they suffer less from inflammatory Lentor, than where they are very rigid and elastic; as commonly happens in the Robust and Laborious, who according to the Observation of *Hippocrates* are most subject to, and suffer most from Inflammations of the Breast and Lungs*.—And this indeed is confirmed by every Day's Experience; and so is likewise the following Remark of the same great Father of Physic, relating to the laudable Expectoration I mentioned above, "Ἅιματι δὲ ξυμμεμιγμένον μὴ πολλῷ πτύελον ζανθὸν, ἐν τοῖσι περιπλευμονικοῖσιν, ἐν ἀρχῇ μὲν τῆς νούσου, πτυόμενον περιεστηκὸν† καὶ κάρτα ὠφελέει": *Hippocr. Prognost.* And indeed it hath been the Observation of the very *Nurses* in some epidemic *Pleuropneumonies* and *Peripneumonies*, that all those who spit Blood do well.—However this is very far from being always true, unless the Matter is conditioned as above: for whenever either very frothy, or sincere florid Blood is spit up, or black and partly coagulated, spongy, liver-coloured Blood, it is quite otherwise; as it shews that there is nothing like Resolution, or Digestion of the obstructing Matter performed; but that, the Obstruction being deeply radicated, and the impelling Force of the Heart vehement, some Vessels are burst open,and an Extravasation

**Coac. Prænot.* 29. *Lib.* II. *Cap.* xvi. *De Pleuritide, Edit. Dureti.*

†So I chuse to read with *Foësius* rather than περιεκτικὼ, as more agreeable to the Sense and the *Hippocratic* Diction.

of Blood made into the Cavities of the Lungs, and so spit up.—For when great Obstructions are formed in some Parts of the Lungs, the Blood must be forced in greater Quantities, and with greater Rapidity, thro' the Vessels that are pervious; which hence, being overdistended, frequently break, and the Blood gushes into the Cavities of the Bronchia, and many Times into the inmost Recesses of the vesicular Cells.—What of this Blood is spit off immediately appears florid and frothy, and does no further Damage; but the chief Misfortune is, that a great Part of it remains commonly in the Lungs, and stuffs up the Air-Bladders, and compresses and obstructs their Blood-vessels; which very much encreases the Difficulty of breathing, and greatly hinders the Circulation of the Blood through the Lungs.—Besides as it is exceeding difficult to be pumped up from these minute vesicular Cells, by continuing there it grows more and more putrid, till at length it becomes a corrosive Sanies, that destroys the very Substance of the Lungs: But of this more hereafter.

As all Inflammations of the Lungs will either quickly choak the Patients by hindering the Passage of the Blood thro' them, or terminate in Suppuration, Gangrene, or Scirrhosity, if the obstructing Matter is not soon kindly resolved, or digested; we should be as early as possible in our Endeavours to abate, and take off, the Inflammation by Bleeding in due Quantities: for when once an Abscess is actually forming, Bleeding can be of no further Service.—Nay when once the *Phlegmon* is too far advanced to be resolved, Bleeding is really disadvantageous, as retarding the next Operation of Nature, to free herself from the offending obstructing Matter, by a kindly Suppuration: For by this Means the Matter is made to stagnate longer, and so grows more and more acrimonious: which at length, by affecting the adjacent Parts, forms a much larger Impostume than would have happened at first, if Nature had been left to her own regular Proceedings; nay many Times it ends in a downright Gangrene, and sometimes in an obstinate Scirrhosity, making the short Remains of Life extreamly miserable.

Physicians note in general, that, after the fourth or fifth Day of a true Peripneumony, Bleeding is of little avail to prevent the Suppuration; for most *Phlegmons* begin to suppurate in that Time, if not resolved before: This will more especially and sooner happen in such a Part as the Lungs, surrounded on all Sides by Warmth and Moisture, and so near the Heart acting on the inflammatory Obstruction with constant and great Force.—So that where the peripneumonic Symptoms continue with great Violence for four or five Days or more successively, an Abscess, or Mortification, is justly to be feared, and little Advantage is to be expected from further Bleeding.

But yet, if either the Pain returns with Violence after having ceased a considerable Time, or seizes another Part of the Breast; it is an Argument that a new Inflammation is forming, which indicates Bleeding as much as the primary, tho' not to the same Degree: for this accessary Seizure being altogether of the same Nature, and on the same *Organ* as the former, requires the same Method to prevent its Advance and further ill Consequences. The Strength of the Patient and Pulse, the Violence of the Pain, and Difficulty of Respiration, are in a great Measure to determine the Quantity: And some Regard must be had also to the Colour and Consistence of the Blood, and the Quantity and Quality of the Serum. I have sometimes ordered Bleeding the ninth or tenth Day from the first Attack, and found the Blood almost as sizy as what was drawn the second or third, and that too where the Lancet had not been timorously used; but the Crassamentum, tho' exceeding tough, was greatly reduced in the Proportion it bore to the Serum.

It is commonly observed, that as soon as this secondary Attack and Pain come on, with any Degree of Violence, the Expectoration, tho' before free and copious, ceases altogether, or is performed with very great Difficulty; the Violence of the Pain not suffering the *Thorax* to be duly expanded, and the Muscles of the Lungs, Breast and Abdomen to act with sufficient Force to eject the Matter: Not to mention that the Inflammation hinders a due Secretion of the lubricating *Mucus*, which should naturally be separated to smooth over the internal Membrane of the *Trachea and Bronchia*, and expedite the Discharge of any matter contained in them.—And we eventually find that, after the Inflammation is abated by Bleeding, the Expectoration returns with Ease and Freedom.

So that tho' in Peripneumonies and Pleuro-peripneumonies you are chiefly to make your Evacuations by Bleeding before the fifth Day; yet on fresh Attacks of violent Pain, difficult Respiration and suppressed Expectoration, you are to begin again, as it were, a-new*, but with great Caution and Moderation: as all Relapses, in these Cases especially, are dangerous, the Sick growing daily weaker and less capable of bearing any considerable Loss of Blood.

* *Hippocrates* bled *Anaxion* the eighth Day, because the Pains continued, and he did not expectorate. *Lib. III. Epid.*

And therefore it will be very imprudent, upon every little Pain, to have Recourse to Bleeding; for more or less Pain continues, particularly after Pleuro-peripneumonies very often, a long Time after the Fever is quite gone off: *Debet prius cessare febris, & postea dolor affecti lateris*, says *Baglivi**.—But Bleeding is, in a peculiar Manner, less proper where a copious Expectoration of laudable Matter goes on pretty easily, tho' it should still continue tinged with Blood, for the Reason I hinted above; *viz.* that it indicates the Resolution and Concoction of the Matter of the new Inflammation. Nay, it is for that very Reason to be avoided, tho' often imprudently ordered, and Astringents stupidly administered, to restrain this slight *Tinge* of Blood: But it is by Persons, who have very little attended to Nature's Operations, and less to *Hippocrates*, her great Interpreter.—It is without all Doubt vastly more proper to alleviate the Pain and Importunity of the Cough by gentle Opiates, cooling, soft, Demulcents, and easy Expectorants.

I have only two Things more to add on the Article of Bleeding in pulmonic Disorders.—The first is, that Bleeding in the *Saphœna*, or Foot, is much less practised in such Cases than might be expected from the Reason of Things, and the certain Experience of its great Efficacy in spitting Blood from the Lungs; I mean after some proper Quantity of Blood may have been drawn from the Arm; *Alexander* the *Trallian*†, many Centuries since, advised it as very useful in that Case.—The second is, that where the Pulse and Strength of the Patient seem not to favour further Blood-letting from a large Vein, and yet the oppressive, laborious, painful Cough and Suffocation remain very urgent; Drawing off Blood by Cupping on the Shoulders, *&c.* may be done with Safety, and frequently gives exceeding great Relief in Disorders of the Breast, as well as of the Head, tho' the Reasons may not be so very obvious and assignable. However it must be considered, that the greater Part of the Blood, drawn this Way, is arterial Blood;—and that the Use of Blisters, Issues, Setons, and even Cupping on those Parts is very notorious in asthmatic Coughs, Defluxions on the Lungs, *&c*; and seems to shew that Revulsions and Evacuations, made this Way, may be very serviceable in Inflammations of the Lungs, and in Event they are so.

Although Bleeding in all Inflammations of the Lungs is indispensably necessary in some Degree, and some Times, when well

* *Prax. medic. Cap. de Pleuritide.*

† *Cap.* vii. *p.* 94. *Ex Edit. Rob. Stephan. Lutetiæ*, 1548. Fol.

timed and executed, quite curative; yet in general there are several other Indications to be answered: For both the Fever, and the particular Inflammation, require a cool diluting Regimen, and nitrous and relaxing Medicines, together with a moderately cool free Air, and as much Quiet as possible both of Body and Mind. It avails little to draw off some of the sizy, obstructing, inflammatory Blood, if the Remainder is not cooled, diluted, and thinned, and a further Generation of the inflammatory Lentor prevented by nitrous Attenuants, cool saponaceous Medicines, diluting, relaxing emollient Drinks, Emulsions, *&c.* which a hot Regimen, hot Medicines, hot Air, much Motion of Body and Agitation of Mind tend greatly to encrease. Persons in asthmatic Paroxysms are under a Necessity of keeping a quiet Posture, and of breathing cool Air, or they are in immediate Danger of Suffocation; how much more so then are these necessary, where there is not only a great Obstruction in the Vessels of the Lungs, but also an Inflammation in their very Substance?—A close, narrow, stifling Room is exceedingly incommodious to any Person sick of a Fever, but much more so to those ill of a Peripneumony, as I have many Times observed, especially among the lower Part of Tradesmen, when two or three Families perhaps live in a House together.—*Celsus*'s Advice is never more proper, nay necessary, in any Kind of Fever than in a peripneumonic, *in amplo conclavi tenendus æger**—If such close Rooms cannot be avoided, they certainly should be frequently, but prudently aired.

Few or no Peripneumonies, or Pleuro-peripneumonies, end well without a free and copious Expectoration; for this is the natural *Crisis* of these Disorders, as hath been noted by *Hippocrates* and all judicious Physicians, and the Want of spitting off the morbid obstructing Matter in a due Manner reckoned extreamly dangerous, Aἱ *ξηραὶ τῶν* | |*λευριτίδων ἄπτυστοι χαλεπώταται*†—And again in the *Prognostic*‖ he says, it is a very bad Symptom when *μηδὲν ἀνακαθαίρηται,—ἀλλὰ πλήρης ἐὼν ζέη ἐν τω φάρυγγι*—The more easy, early and large the concoted Expectoration is, so much the better.—Indeed generally at the Begining it is crude and thin, but soon becomes of a whitish yellow Colour and greater Consistence, when Matters proceed rightly; and about the third Day it is

* *Lib. III. Cap.* vii.

† *Coac. Prænot.* 3. *Cap.* xvi. *Edit. Dureti.*

‖ *Sect.* xiii. *Edit. Linden.*

commonly streaked with Blood, or the Blood is so incorporated with it as to give it a bloody *Tinge, flavo-rubescens* as *Baglivi** calls it, or in the *Hippocratic Phrase*, Πτύελου ὕραιμον.—This Kind of Matter, when freely spit off, gives great Relief to the Respiration, Pain and Oppression at the Breast, and generally terminates the Disease in seven Days.

But nothing more effectually promotes Expectoration (by attenuating and resolving the impacted Matter) than drinking freely and frequently of cooling, relaxing, and gently saponaceous Diluents; such an thin Whey, the *Barley Ptisan* with Liquorice, Figs, *&c.* the Decoction, or rather Infusion of the *pectoral Herbs*, as Ground-ivy, Maiden-hair, Colts-foot, Hyssop, *&c.*—There should be gently acidulated with Juice of Lemon, or Sevil-orange:—if any Thing more detergent is wanting to the above Drinks, *Honey* may be added: An admirable, natural, cordial *Sapo*, thrown almost out of the modern *Materia Medica* I know not why, nor how; for where it gripes or purges one, it agrees with a thousand, and even its griping and purging Quality may be easily corrected by boiling.—*Hippocrates* used *Oxymel* and *Mulsum* in such Cases, and advises against drinking mere Water in pulmonic Fevers, as neither good for the Cough, nor to promote Expectoration†:—Any or all of these Things, by Turns, drank warm answer the above Intention exceedingly well, if taken in frequent but small Draughts, sipping them as it were perpetually; for by this Means much of the relaxing, resolving Vapor is also drawn into the Lungs, and much probably absorbed by their imbibing Vessels; so that relaxing and diluting is thus carried on in a double Manner, and of Course very effectually. Very large Draughts should not be taken at once; for they overcharge the Stomach, produce Indigestion and Flatulence, and force up the Midriff too much, which greatly embarrasses the Respiration:—Therefore *Hippocrates* advises to drink in those Diseases out of a Cup with a narrow Mouth||, probably both that the Liquor and Vapor might be preserved warm longer, and that less might be drank at a Time, and also that the Steam might be more copiously carried into the Mouth and Nose.—However still he advises to

* *Cap. de Pleuritide.*

† *De Vict. in Morb. acut. Sect.* xxx. *Edit. Linden.*

|| Μὴ ψυχρὸν, ὀλίγον δὲ ἐκ Βομβυλίου οὐκ ἐυρυστομου; *for so it should be read, or simply* Βομβυλίου. *as all the Commentators agree, Lib. III. de Morbis. Sect.* xxiv. *Edit. Linden. See* Galen, Erotian, *and* Foësius, *on the Word* Βομβυλιος.

drink freely to promote the Expectoration, without which the Patient dies* :—And many Kinds of Drinks he advises for this Purpose, but particularly recommends Barley-water, Honey and Water, Oxymel, and Vinegar and Water.

These relaxing emollient Drinks and Vapors are in a more especial Manner necessary, when the Expectoration is very difficult and tough, and for those of a *strigose* Habit of Body and very rigid Fibres; such as hard labouring People, and those of a hot and dry Constitution, generally are. For as a very dry Air, whether cold or hot, is found to hinder a free and copious Expectoration; a moist and warm† one cannot but promote it, by relaxing the Vessels, and attenuating also in some Degree the over viscid Humors.—*Baglivi*‖ greatly recommends the *fervida potio* for resolving pulmonic Obstructions, but I think a moderate Degree of Warmth is more proper both for resolving and relaxing.—Fomentations applied too hot on the external Parts are found to incrassate the Humors, and corrugate the Skin, and are vastly improper upon inflamed Parts.—The Vapors may be made more or less stimulating, or relaxing, as the Case requires.—I have known the Fumes of Vinegar itself of no small Service in malignant Peripneumonies: Several Kinds of Medicines may undoubtedly be administered with great Advantage by Way of Vapor: The Steam of *camphorated Vinegar* is no contemptible Thing in many Cases.

Hippocrates and the Ancients were so sensible of the Necessity of Expectoration in pulmonic Disorders, that they not only endeavour to promote it, by the Means I have mentioned; but also in difficult Cases used much more powerful Expectorants§ : The Cream of Barley with Honey of Oil, Oxymel, Hyssop, Rue, Galbamum, Mustard, Pepper, *Silphium*** were some of the milder: in desperate Cases white Hellebore,‡ Elaterium, *Ἄνθος χαλκοῦ* were advised: and desperate indeed they must be to be justified now-a-days; but as

* *Lib. I. de Morbis, Sect.* xxvi.—*De Locis in Homine, Sect.* xxx. xxxvii. *Edit. Lindeni, and in many other Places.*

† Aretæus *says, neither cold Drink nor cold Air are good in Pleurisies.*

‖ *De Pleuritide.*

§ *Ἰσχυρότατα ἐπαναχρεμπτήρια φάρμακα*; *De Locis in Homine Sect.* xxx. *Edit. Linden.*

** *Lib. III. de Morbis, Sect,* xviii, xxv. *Edit. Linden, & alibi passim; and* Aretæus *advises much the same Things in Pleurisies and Peripneumonies.*

‡ *Lib. III. de Morbis, Sect.* xvii. *Ed. Linden.*

they had then no other, desperate Remedies were to be tried in desperate Diseases.—We have a much more ample *Materia Medica*, and can avail ourselves of Things of a much gentler Nature.—But I have several Times given an Emetic in Peripneumonies with great Advantage, when the Expectoration hath been suddenly suppressed, and the Difficulty of Breathing greatly augmented; but it was when a proper Quantity of Blood had been drawn antecedently, and the Violence of the Fever abated: but in such Cases very little should be drank after it to promote the Vomiting. *Oxymel scilliticum*, frequently doth great Service this Way, and its Virtues in relieving asthmatic Disorders are notorious: It not only, in a proper Dose, pukes gently, but is also an excellent cooling Attenuant, and useful *Eccoprotic*, and a very good Diuretic: it is undoubtedly greatly superior to simple Oxymel, and may be so blended with oleaginous emollient Medicines as to be highly serviceable, as an easy Expectorant.—Where very soft, demulcent lubricating Medicines are indicated, our common *Linctus* of *Sperma ceti, Ol. amygdal. dulc*, or cold drawn *Linseed-oil* with *Syrup. althææ, Papav. errat. diacodium*, or the like, answer the Intention.—But where Oils disagree, a Mucilage of Quince-seeds, or Linseed with *Rob* of Elder-berries, or black, Currants, or their Syrup, or that of Poppies, is very useful and grateful.—*Nitre*, that very necessary, cooling Attenuant, is very agreeably administered in either of these Compositions; and perhaps *Camphire*, given this Way, is the least nauseous.—The utmost Care should be taken never to give strong Expectorants in the Begining of Peripneumonies, till proper Bleeding, *&c.* may have allayed the Impetuosity of the Blood and Fever; otherwise they will encrease the Inflammation and Danger of Suffocation, and eventually intercept what they were designed to pump up: The Matter should be first concocted, and then expectorated.—Another Thing is also necessary to be observed in the Use of such Expectorants as *Oxymel scilliticum*, oily Medicines, gummose Mixtures, and pectoral Decoctions; and that is, that we do not bring on any considerable Purging, which will certainly suppress the Expectoration, and endanger the Life of the Patient.

Though a free Expectoration of concocted Matter is of the highest Service in the Cure of Peripneumonies and Pleuroperipneumonies, and should be always encouraged; yet there are some Kinds of Expectoration of very *ill Omen.*—It is particularly a very ill Sign, when much sincere florid, or frothy Blood is spit up, and thus it is pronounced by *Hippocrates* and *Aretæus*; though they both speak so favourably of the concocted Matter that is expectorated with a bloody *Tinge*: The former condemn the || *τύελον λίην αἱματῶδες* *, the later the *Δίαιμον ἀνθηρὸν σφόδρα*; nay *Aretæus* says, Ἐ*στί το Δίαιμον τῶν ἄλλων κάκιον* †, and I think so too for the Reason above-mentioned; for this fresh frothy Blood proceeds from a Rupture of Arteries in the Lungs, and not from a Resolution of the inflammatory Obstruction. Now, if Arteries are burst in the Lungs, the Blood gushes into the Cavities of the Bronchia, sometimes in such Quantities as to cause a sudden Suffocation, if not immediately brought up: but more commonly it leaks into the pulmonary Vesiculæ, and many Times Vessels are broke in the inmost Recesses of the Lungs, Part of which may indeed be soon spit up fresh and florid, but much is very apt to remain in the ultimate Ramifications, and cellular Interstices of the Bronchia; which stuffs up the Lungs, compresses the surrounding Blood-Vessels, and at length putrefies and corrodes all around it: Hence a speedy Suffocation, a dangerous *Vomica*, or a direct Gangrene frequently ensues.—This extravasated Matter also may indeed be partly spit off in the Form of a bloody *Sanies*, or of livid and black Concretions; but it is commonly with such Difficulty, and so violent a Cough, as even to encrease the Extravasation: But it is generally so imperfectly, that much remains in the Lungs, and produces most fatal Consequences. *Hippocrates* || therefore declares such a Kind of Expectoration exceeding dangerous; and truly it is most commonly a Sign of an impending Mortification, or one actually formed.—I remember many Years since to have observed a Matter spit up at the Close of a Peripneumony, by one Mr. *Clark*, a Master of a Merchantship of this Town, which exactly resembled Pieces of boiled Spleen, or rather more spongy, some of which were very fœtid: He died the 19th Day of the Disease. This corresponds with a Prognostic of *Baglivi* § from *Dodonæus: Qui spuunt sanguinem nigrum porosum**. ad instar spongiæ, iis pars aliqua sphacelo correpta est in pulmone, & omnes pereunt.*

As soon therefore as this Expectoration of florid Blood appears,

* *Coac. Prænot.* 17. *Lib. II. Cap. xvi. de Pleuritid. &c. ex Edit. Dureti.*

† *Cap. de Pulmonaria.*

|| *Prognostic.—Coac. Prænot.* 45. *Cap. de Pleuritid ex Edit. Duret.*

§ *Vid Baglivi Opera, Lugduni* 1704, 4*to. p.* 87.

** Αἱματος θρομβους μελανας. *Hippocr, Lib. III. de Morbis Sect.* xix. *Edit. Linden.*

I immediately direct Bleeding in such Quantities, as are adapted to the Strength of the Patient; in order to abate the too rapid Motion of the Blood, lessen the Inflammation, and prevent as much as possible the further Effusion of Blood amongst the pulmonic Vesiculæ and Cellules, where it would do infinite Mischief.—If the *Hæmoptoë* continues, Bleeding in the *Saphæna* will be found of the utmost Service.—Besides this, cooling Emulsions, nitrous, demulcent, mucilaginous Medicines, vegetable Acids, and even mineral, if the *Hæmoptoë* be very considerable, are required: A Decoction of red Poppies, Colts-foot and Figs, acidulated with Elixir of Vitriol, makes an admirable Drink in such Cases:—And we must endeavour to moderate the Violence of the Cough by *Diacodium*, a soft Linctus, or the like.—But I utterly disapprove of strong Astringents, and large Doses of Opiates, as I have often known the imprudent Use of them, in such Circumstances, bring on a vast *Orthopnœa*, and most terrible Symptoms: For the extravasated Blood must be ultimately spit off, or the Patient never recovers; but this is impossible without more or less of a Cough to pump it up.—I have several Times known very large Impostumations happen after such Kind of Peripneumonies, where the Patient had survived the Fever for several Days, nay for some Weeks.

Though a morbid *Viscosity* commonly prevails in pulmonic Fevers, yet there are not a few, in which an acrid *Tenuity* is predominant.—And as we observe in *Ophthalmics*, the *Defluxion* sometimes as thick as *Glew*, sometimes as thin as *Water*, and sharp as *Brine*, fretting the very Skin of the Cheeks as it trickles down; so the Matter expectorated in some Peripneumonies is extreamly thin and crude, and the Defluxion so very acrid as to excoriate the Wind-pipe, *&c.* and cause an incessant and very violent Cough.

The sharp thin Humors, in catarrhal Fevers, very often bring on peripneumonic Symptoms, by causing a constant Irritation and Agitation of the Lungs; and no small Mischief likewise arises from the violent Concussions, that are occasioned by the frequent *Sneezing*, which commonly attend such acrid *Catarrhs*, which are sometimes so *virulent* as to inflame the Nostrils, and blister the very Lips.—The great Father of Physic, in his *most admirable Prognostic*, hath pronounced it very dangerous when *Catarrhs* and *Sneezing* precede, or supervene peripneumonic Diseases.—I once knew very severe pleuropneumonic Pains immediately brought on by a Fit of Sneezing, after they had quite ceased for a very considerable Time.

In this *catarrhal Peripneumony*, if I may so term it, no great

Loss of Blood is necessary; some however should be drawn, in the Begining, to abate the present inflammatory Disposition, and prevent future ill Accidents. Blisters also should be applied early, to avert and draw off the acrid Defluxion: And here even gentle Purgatives are proper to carry off the serous *Colluvies.* The Author of the second Book *de Morbis*, amongst the *Hippocratic* Writings*, advises to purge in an *Erysipelas* of the Lungs, where the Expectoration is large and thin: And I have frequently experienced the good Effect of Purgatives in these catarrhal Peripneumonies, though they are utterly improper in those that are attended with a laudable concocted Expectoration. Much less Drink is necessary in this Peripneumony than in the dry Kind; some *demulcent pectoral Ptisan* however is proper to temperate the Acrimony of the Humors, and should be taken warm with some mild Diaphoretics, to promote easy breathing Sweats: *Coffee* in this Case is both a pleasant and a profitable Drink. Some gentle Opiates likewise are required to moderate the Cough, such as Diacodium, or *Elixir Asthmaticum*, not in large Doses, but frequently repeated; with which may be joined Spermaceti, Myrrh, Olibanum, and Camphire, as they will also tend to incrassate the thin catarrhal Humor, and abate its Irritation; which, as *Hippocrates* says, brings on Peripneumonies, *&c.* which cease as soon as the Defluxion becomes more thick and concocted. †

But of much worse Omen, than this thin crude Expectoration, is the *livid, gleety*, and *sanious*, frequently resembling the *Leys of red Wine*, sometimes more *black*, and sometimes very *fœtid*; for this either proceeds from a gangrenous State of the Lungs, or from a Destruction of the Crasis of the Blood by very great Acrimony, which is often the Case in the highly scorbutic: A vast many Instances of which we have lately had amongst the *Sailors*, after long Cruises and *West-India Expeditions.*—The Blood drawn from such Peripneumonies appeared in a dissolving putrescent State; the *Crassamentum* loose and tender, the *Serum* turbid and reddish: The black Tongue, and Teeth furred with a dark thick *Sordes*, the offensive Breath, and high-coloured, or blackish rank Urine, which were generally observed, denoted a great Corruption of the Humors; and the black Spots, or bloody Dysentery, which frequently appeared the fifth, sixth, or seventh Day, more strongly

* *Sect.* liii. *Edit. Linden.*

† *De veteri Medicina, Sect.* xxxiii. *Edit. Linden.*

evinced it.—It was surprising how much the Pulse and Strength of the Patient sunk after Bleeding in such Cases: With no small Concern and Astonishment I several Times observed a vast Anxiety, Fainting, cold Sweat, and a thready intermitting Pulse, very soon succeed it; though at the very Begining of the Fever, and when the Pulse seemed strong and throbbing before.—I have seen this even in Pleuro-peripneumonies, where the Pain of the Side was violent, the Load at Breast great, and the Cough considerable; otherwise the peripneumonic Appearance might have been imagined to be a mere Symptom of a malignant Fever.—I am very sure this putrid Peripneumony never bore a second Bleeding with Advantage, seldom indeed the first, unless there was some considerable Degree of *Firmness* and *Tension* in the Pulse*.—When I was diffident as to Bleeding, I ordered Scarification and Cupping sometimes with Success; though in one or two Cases, the Effusion from the Scarifications was vastly profuse, and could not be totally restrained, till the Patient expired.

Here then some *anti-putrescent* pectoral Medicines are necessary; a Decoction of Figs, Colts-foot, and red Poppies, well acidulated with Juice of Sevil-orange, or Lemon first and then with *Gas Sulphuris*, or *Elixir Vitrioli*, is very proper.—Nitre, *Olibanum*, Myrrh, Flowers of Sulphur and Bole may be administered with *Conserv. Lujulæ, Rob* of Elder or Currants, Mucilage of Quince-seeds, and *Syrup. de Rubo Idæo: Camphorated Vinegar* with Syrup of Elder and Rasberries is an excellent Medicine; a Spoonful or two of these latter should be given ever and anon. Sound *Cyder*, and Wine and Water with Sevil-orange or Lemon Juice, drank warm, promote Expectoration when deficient, and correct the *alcalescent Acrimony*.—Tincture of Roses with red Poppy Flowers, moderated an inordinate Defluxion of the thin bloody *Ichor*; frequently however *Oxymel scillit. & Aq. Cinnamom. fort.* were necessary to pump up the Matter, when a great Rattling in the Wind-pipe, and Difficulty of Breathing, indicated a vast Quantity of it in the Lungs: And yet very often the Importunity and Violence of the Cough was to be appeased by *Elixir asthmaticum, Diacodium, &c.*—Sago, Panado, Jelly of Hartshorn, roasted Apple, Cream of Barley, or thick Gruel with a little Wine and Juice of Lemon, given little at a Time, but often, were necessary to support the Patient; even Strawberries, Rasberries, Currants, Cherries, were sometimes indulged

* *Vid. Obs. nostr. de Aere, &c. Vol. II. Jan. Febr.* 1746.

with Advantage. Nor is this a new Practice; for *Aretæus** advises the Fruits of the Season, such as Figs, *&c.* in the Cure of Pleurisies; and the same Author very justly says, that Food may be so adapted, as to be made Physic†.—I have been more large in the dietetic Part; for in a Word a proper Support of the Patients, and gaining Time till the Acrimony of the Humors was corrected, and the Lungs disburthened from the putrid Colluvies, seemed to be the great Affair; at the Close, at least, the whole depended on a well-regulated Diet, in which Toast with diluted red Port-wine, mulled up with Sevil-orange Rind, Mace, or Cinnamon, and well acidulated, were remarkably useful.—I seldom found Blisters of any Service in this Case, often indeed mischievous, fretting much, and venting a vast Deal of thin bloody Matter, and sometimes attended with Mortifications.

A very thin yellow Spitting, as if tinged with Saffron, is another ill Symptom in pneumonic Fevers; as either denoting that the inflammatory Lentor sticks fast in the Arteries of the Lungs, and that nothing, but the serous and thinnest Part of the Blood, is strained through them; or else it shews that the whole Mass of Blood begins to dissolve, and its bilious Principles to be highly exalted, and that all tends to a general Putrefaction.—In very putrid Fevers even the Milk, Sweat, *&c.* turn yellow, and stagnant Blood putrefying and dissolving always puts on that Appearance.—*Hippocrates* indeed commends that Expectoration, in which the *yellow* is strongly mixed with the *Spittle* ‖ (or an intimate Mixture of yellow with white); but then he declares the *Sincere yellow Spit* (*ξανθὸν ἄκρητον* †) dangerous; and it is constantly found so, and is commonly attended with a violent Cough, and brought up with exceeding great Difficulty: Besides, it is many Times succeeded by an *Hæmoptoë* from a Rupture of the Vessels; and this particularly when the Tongue appears very red, dry, smooth, and shining, with a Kind of *livid Bladders*** at the Top*; which, by the Way, is a bad Symptom in all Kinds of Fevers.—It is carefully to be distinguished

* *De curatione Pleuritidis.*

† Ἐν Τροφῇ *γὰρ κείσεται τὰ φὰρμακα, ἀτὰρ καὶ τά φάρμακὰ ἡ* Τροφῇ. *Ibid.*

‖ Τὸ *ξανθὸν ξυμμεμιγμένον ἰσχυρῶς τῶ πτυέλω.Prognostic. Sect.* xiii. *Edit. Linden.*

† *Ibid.*

** Πομφόλυξ *ὑποπέλιος on the Tongue* Hippocrates *pronounces dangerous, and that it precedes Spitting of Blood.* Coac. Prænot. 6. Cap. de pleuritide.

in Practice, from which of the above Causes this thin bilious Expectoration proceeds; in order to which we should diligently consider the Pulse, State of the Blood, and Temper of the Body: for very different Indications will arise from the different Causes.

I shall conclude these Remarks, on the Expectoration in pulmonic Fevers, with the following Observations of the great *Hippocrates.*—"Matter should be spit off easily and early in Peripneumonies and Pleurisies; the Colour of it should be a yellow well mixed with the Spittle, or a concocted yellow Matter that is tinged with some, but not too much, Blood:—If this happens in the Begining of the Disease, it is very advantageous; but is not so much to be depended upon after the seventh Day.—It is exceeding bad when there seems a great Quantity, and Rattling, of Matter in the Throat, and yet nothing is spit off. It is indeed, in all Cases, dangerous when nothing is expectorated; but that which is very viscid, small, and globular, or frothy, is unprofitable. The sincere yellow unmixed Spitting is bad; when very bloody, or livid, it is dangerous; especially when this Appearance is very early; but that which is quite black is worst of all: It is an ill Sign also when it is very green (*ἴωδες*). Whatever is spit up with great Difficulty, violent Cough, and no Relief to the Pain and Oppression, shews the Case to be bad." See *Coac. Prænotion.* 13, 14, 14, 15, 17, 18. *Edit. Dureti, Cap. de Pleuritide*, compared with the *Prognostic of Hippocrates*; who says, a concocted Expectoration is like good *Pus**, not thin and gleety, nor very yellow, very bloody, green, or livid: Indeed in any Abscess, or Ulcer, such Colours are of very ill Omen, as denoting a high Degree of Acrimony.

But when a Resolution, or Concoction of the inflammatory Obstructions of the Lungs happens, not only Part is thrown into the Cavities of the *Bronchia*, and so spit off; but also Part of it passes on into the corresponding Veins, and thence moves on with the rest of the Blood, in the common Road of Circulation; till at length it is partly carried off by thick turbid Urine, in large Quantities, depositing much reddish, yellow-coloured Sediment, which in peripneumonic Disorders always betokens Good, and partly also sometimes by bilious Stools.—*Hippocrates* observes, that this thick subsiding reddish Urine in Pleurisies is a secure Sign†, and that it carries off

* Πέπονα δὲ ἐσί τὰ μὲν Πτύελα, ὁκόταν γένηται ὅμοια τῷ Πύω. *De Vict. acut. Sect.* liii. *Edit. Lindeni.*

† 586 *Coac. Prænot. Edit. Foësii.*

Peripneumonies when thick and plentiful*.—He describes these concocted Urines as having ὑποστάσιας ὑπερύθρους ὁκοῖον Ὄροβος†, that is, a Kind of a pale lateritious Sediment, as we call it.—But he justly observes, it is an exceeding ill Symptom, if, from being before thick, they grow thin about the fourth Day||;—and so it is indeed at any Time of the Disease, whilst the Fever continues very considerable.

Nothing promotes these Urines and Stools more effectually than emollient laxative Clysters, as they are a Kind of Fotus, and gentle Stimulant, to all the Parts of the lower Belly, and not only tend to discharge Urine and Stool, but Wind also, which sometimes, by huffing up the Abdomen and Midriff, greatly straiten the Respiration.—Besides when the gross Excrements press on the Bottom of the *Aorta*, and Heads of the *Iliacs;* too much Blood regurgitates to the superior Parts, particularly the Breast, which encreases the Inflammation, Oppression, *&c.*—*Hippocrates* therefore advises § cooling Clysters in peripneumonic Fevers, especially the first three Days**; and *Aretæus* says, we should inject an acrid Clyster, in some Cases, when we cannot well bleed‡.—The greatest Care however should be taken not to throw the Patient into a profuse Diarrhoea, which will suppress the Expectoration without relieving the Disease; and accordingly the great Oracle of Physic†† says, it is a bad Symptom where it happens to Pleuritics and Peripneumonics; because when there is a great Flux of Humors downwards, the superior Parts grow dry, the Spitting ceases, and the Sick die§§: So that the Body should not be too costive, which would encrease the Fever; nor too loose ‡‡, lest the Spitting and Strength of the Patient fail.—This is *Hippocratic* Physic, and I am sure as rational, and well founded, as any of the modern.—But to proceed.

Sometimes the morbid Matter is critically translated to the

**De Vict. acut. Sect* liii. *Ed. Linden.*

† *Ibid.*

|| *Coac, Prænot.* 53. *Cap. de. Pleuritid.*—20. *Cap, de Urinis, Edit. Dureti.*

§ *De Affect. Sect.* viii. *Edit. Linden.*

** *De Vict. acut. Sect.* lii. *Edit. Linden.*

‡ *De curatione Pulmonar.*

†† *Hippocrat. Aphorism. 16. Sect.* i.

§§ *Lib. III. de Morb. Sect. xvii. Ed. Linden.*

‡‡ *Ibid.*

lower Parts, producing Phlegmons, Impostumes, erysipelatose or œdematous Swellings, Ulcers, *&c*; particularly in Persons formerly subject to swoln or sore Legs, which are frequently noted to swell, or break up again, at the Close of peripneumonic Disorders, to the great Relief of the Breast. It is a well known Thing, that on drying up Ulcers in the Legs suddenly, the Lungs become forthwith affected; and that hydropic Tumors of these Parts, forced up by laced Stockings, Bandage, *&c.* immediately bring on asthmatic Disorders: Which sufficiently shew the natural Consent there is between the Breast and lower Parts, and that they are reciprocally affected by Disorders.—Wherefore it seems rational, in severe pulmonic Disorders, to attempt a Derivation of the Humors to the Legs by tepid Bathing, Blisters, *&c*: and in Fact this hath been often practised with Success.—How often do we find a *Metastasis* of the Gout to the Lungs suddenly relieved by a *Revulsion* of it to the Feet by acrid Cataplasms? Where there is great Danger, we should neglect nothing.—When Blisters, applied to the Legs in pulmonic Diseases, ulcerate severely, they commonly give great Relief; but they are often exceeding difficult to be healed up.—This was particularly remarkable in the Years 1740—41—46—47*.—I then also observed, that if the Discharge, from the ulcerated Blisters, was suddenly suppressed; not only the Cough and Difficulty of Breathing returned, but sometimes a very great Purging, and sometimes very profuse Sweats forthwith came on: So that, in not a few Cases, the Patient was either worn out by the Pain and vast Discharge from the Blisters, or run down by a colliquative Diarrhœa, or Sweat; terrible *Aphthæ* frequently closing the fatal Scene.—Probably this arose from the great Acrimony of the Lymph and Serum, which have been jellied as it were by the preceding Fever, and now dissolving, was turned into a Kind of putrid *Ichor* (for when *Serum* is coagulated by Heat, its next State is a putrid *Liquamen*, or Dissolution): Nor did it only issue in profuse Stools and Sweats, but vented itself likewise by other Ways, as very Foul, sharp, turbid Urine, pustular Eruptions, angry Boils, watery Bladders, very painful and fretting, on several Parts of the Body; as the Shoulders, Arms, Back, Breast, *&c.*—From some Observations of this Kind, it is likely the Ancients (who always carefully studied to follow and second Nature's Endeavours) applied *acrid Epithems*, as Salt, Mustard, *&c.* to the Breast, Back and Shoulders, in pulmonic Distempers. It is

* *Vid. Obs. nostr. de Aere & Morb. Epidem. Vol. II.*

certain there is a great Consent between the Skin and the Lungs, as is evident in a repelled Itch, Small-pox, Measles, *&c.* which immediately fall on the Breast.—Therefore blistering the above Parts, after a proper Quantity of Blood is drawn off, should seem a rational Practice, especially towards the Decline of peripneumonic Fevers.

Though Nature takes sometimes these different Methods of relieving herself in peripneumonic Diseases, yet her proper and common Effort is by Expectoration; and while that proceeds well, we may indeed favour her Attempt, but never interrupt it, which violent Purging, Sweating, and the like, will infallibly do:—So that those other, just now mentioned, seem only the By-ways of Nature, and the morbific Matter is then only to be strongly solicited through them, when the high Road is either stopped, or greatly embarrassed.

CHAP. III.

Of the Peripneumonia notha.

WHAT I have said above relates to the Nature and Management of inflammatory, or true Peripneumonies; but there is a Disease, noted chiefly by *Sydenham*, and the later Authors, under the Name of a *Peripneumonia notha*, in which, though the Load at Breast is very great, the Breathing very difficult, and the Cough very importunate, and sometimes violent, (all sufficiently denoting the Lungs to be considerably affected) yet the Fever and Heat are small, many Times scarce perceptible, the Pulse either quick, weak, and small, or sluggish and oppressed, never hard and tense.—So that as this Distemper hath very different, and almost quite contrary Symptoms to those of a true Peripneumony in several Respects; it is reasonable to suppose it arises from very different Causes, and requires a very different Method of Cure.—And in Fact we see, that bastard Peripneumonies commonly seize the old and phlegmatic, the weak and lax, the fat and unwieldy, and are most rife in wet, flabby, foggy Weather and Winter Seasons; whereas the true inflammatory Peripneumony generally attacks the robust, vigorous and active, and is most frequent in cold, dry Weather, during north-east Winds, and high Stations of the Barometer.—These two Diseases then seem to differ almost as much as ardent and slow nervous Fevers; or as much as an inflammatory Quinsy doth from one that is purely humoral, or arising merely from a serous Defluxion.—And such a serous acrid *Colluvies* may fall on the Lungs, be diffused into and amongst the inmost Recesses of their vesicular and cellular Cavities, and occasion a great Oppression on, and some Degree of Obstruction in, the pulmonic and bronchial Arteries, and so greatly hinder a regular Circulation of the Blood through the Lungs. The frequent Chills and Flushes of Heat however, the Quickness and Irregularity of the Pulse, Anxiety and Weight at Breast, Pain and Giddiness of the Head, Foulness of the Tongue, *&c.* sufficiently indicate a feverish Habit.

Upon the whole, this Disease seems to have its Origin from a *pituitous Lentor* of the Blood, and a *ropy* Disposition of the *Lymph* and *Serum*; which being greatly redundant from suppressed Perspiration, *&c.* and put in Motion by a febrile Heat, or sudden Agitation of the Humors, is thrown on the Lungs faster than it can pass off (for viscid Humors never pass as freely through the Extremities of the Arteries as when more thin and fluxile;) whence, being there more and more congested, it more and more obstructs the pulmonic Vessels, till at last a fatal Stagnation ensues, and Death the Consequence.—We see this exemplified, in a particular Manner, by bringing on an artificial Peripneumony, if I may so call it; *viz.* Let a Girl labouring under a *leucophlegmatic Chlorosis* (where such a heavy viscous *Pituita*, as I have mentioned, predominates) be forced into great and long continued Exercise; her Lungs at length become so stuffed and loaded, that she falls into a vast Difficulty of Breathing, and even an entire Suffocation.—This hath really happened in several instances, where the Exercise hath been pushed too far.—I might have taken Notice also, that such a pituitous Lentor of the Blood and Humors doth not give off a sufficient Quantity of animal Spirits, to actuate the Vessels with Force enough to carry on a due Circulation.

As there are many intermediate States, between the violent inflammatory Peripneumony, and this last mentioned, no distinct settled Method of Cure can be laid down; because the peripneumonic Malady, to be immediately treated of, may sometimes incline much more to the inflammatory State, and sometimes much less.

For a Disease is a Disorder in the animal Œconomy, distinguished indeed by such and such particular Symptoms, and called by such or such a Name; but each particular Disease, in every individual Patient, is to be considered by the attending Physician, not according to the *Nomenclature,* but according to the Nature, Causes and Symptoms of the particular Disease in that particular Person; and Measures should be taken accordingly.—Thus if I meet with a great Load and Uneasiness at Breast, a difficult hot Breathing, Cough, *&c.* with a full, strong, quick Pulse, or a very tense and hard one, in a strong and vigorous Person; I have a sufficient Warranty to be much more free and frequent in Bleeding, than where the Oppression, Cough, *&c.* are not attended with such a rapid and strong, or quick and tense Pulse; especially if I previously knew the labouring Person to be of a weak, lax, or phlegmatic Constitution.

So that when the Pulse is weak and low, the Heat little, or not considerably above the natural, the Urine pale and crude, and so on; I must proceed with great Caution in bleeding a pulmonic Patient, though the Load and Oppression at Breast may be very urgent.—And in Event when Blood is drawn from a Person under a bastard Peripneumony, it either appears loose, thin and florid, or more commonly of a darkish livid Hue, and not coated over with a thick viscid *Buff,* as in common Inflammations of the Lungs.—And it is observable that the Patient soon sinks, and grows considerably weaker after such an Evacuation, though, for the present, seemingly relieved, as to the Anxiety and Load on the *Prœcordia:* For as Bleeding, in this Case especially, weakens the Powers of Nature, and the Action of the Solids on the Fluids; the morbific Lentor, the continent Cause of the Disease, is thereby encreased.—Of this *Sydenham* himself was so sensible, that he particularly cautions against repeated Bleedings in a *Peripneumonia notha,* especially in Persons of a gross Habit of Body, and that had passed the Flower of their Age*; though in a true Peripneumony, he imagined he could as effectually *vent* the Matter of the Disease through the *Orifice of a Vein,* as by the *Trachea itself* †.—It is moreover certain, that common *catarrhal Fevers,* in which a serous *Colluvies* abounds, will not bear very large Bleeding, much less a *Peripneumonia notha,* where a slimy *Pituita* is redundant.

But as Bleeding, on the one Hand, is to be used with great

* *Cap. de Peripneumonia notha.*

† *Cap. de Pleuritids.*

Caution in this Disorder, so on the other are very heating and stimulating Medicines, especially at the Begining of the Distemper; otherwise not only the Oppression on the Breast is greatly encreased, but a comatose Disposition also is readily brought on. For the morbid Lentor may be forced in too great Quantities on the Vessels of the Brain, and accumulated there, as well as in the Lungs; and evidently is so from the Giddiness, Pain and Heaviness of the Head, which commonly attend the bastard Peripneumony: For as the free Descent of the Humors from the Head is considerably hindered by the too great Repletion of, and almost Stagnation in, the Lungs; the right Ventricle of the Heart hath not sufficient Room to play off its Contents of Blood; and receive others freely.

We should proceed therefore with great Circumspection in treating these Kinds of Diseases, which are always dangerous, and frequently fatal; and the more so, as, at the Begining, the Mildness of the Symptoms is too apt to mislead both the Patient, and less cautious, or unexperienced Physician, into too great a Neglect, or wrong Management. I have seen it more than once, or twice, taken for a mere Fit of *Hypochondriacism*, where a very few Hours have shewn the fatal Mistake.—But where a perpetual laborious Wheezing, great Anxiety and constant Oppression on the *Præcordia*, comatose Symptoms, cold Extremities, and dark lead-coloured Nails and Visage are come on; the Physician must be more stupid than the Patient, not to see the immediate Danger.

I think in general more or less Blood should be drawn in the Begining; but, as *Sydenham* well observes*, during the Operation let the Patient be kept in a recumbent Posture, by which means Faintness, otherwise very apt to come on, will be avoided.—For this not only lessens the too great Load and Distension of the Vessels, but also makes Room for such Drinks and Medicines as may be necessary in the Process of the Cure: But as to the Repetition of Bleeding we should be very cautious, and well consider the State of the Blood, the Strength of the Pulse and Patient, before we advise it. It is undoubtedly sometimes necessary.—We are frequently obliged to bleed repeatedly in asthmatic Paroxysms, where there is no Manner of Fever.—Mild, attenuant, saponaceous Medicines, thin diluting detergent Drinks, and the Application of Blisters should succeed Bleeding: An Infusion of inciding, deterging, pectoral Herbs, as Ground-ivy, Hyssop, Penny-royal, Liquorice, or a thin Mustard-

* *De Peripneumonia notha.*

whey sweetened with Honey, and sharpened with Lemon, are proper for common Drink.—Some Dilution is necessary in this Disease, though nothing so much as in a true Peripneumony, nor indeed doth Nature call for it by any great Thirst; yet as the Lentor, predominant in this Disorder, is most readily dissolved by warm watery Liquors, some are undoubtedly proper.

As a bastard Peripneumony is commonly attended with frequent Urgings to vomit, I think it pretty clearly hints to us the Expediency of relieving Nature that Way; and accordingly I have often experienced the good Effects of gentle Vomits in it, after some Blood had been drawn off.—A Spoonful or two of *Oxymel scilliticum, or Vinum Ipecacoanhæ,* with a few Draughts of Mustard-whey, or the like, are sufficient: A large Quantity of any Kind of Liquor should not be drank.—This not only pumps up much heavy *Pituita* from the Stomach and Lungs, but also, by the Concussion it gives the whole vascular System, promotes a general Attenuation and Fluxility of the Humors; and a Stool, or Sweat commonly succeeds.

The mighty Cures, in Pleurisies, *&c.* boasted of by *Rulandus**, and others with the *antimonial Aqua benedicta,* were greatly owing to its emetic Quality; and the famous Poudre *des chartreux* †, or *Kermes mineral,* gained such high Repute in Pleurisies, Peripneumonies and Defluxions on the Breast, in a great Measure at least, from the gentle Efforts it creates to vomit.—Undoubtedly it hath had good Effects in catarrhal Fevers, and pituitous Peripneumonies; but to give either the one or the other in inflammatory Peripneumonies, or Pleurisies, without previous Bleeding, is utterly wrong, dangerous and empirical.

Let me here take Notice of what I many Years ago mentioned, that the best of all the antimonial Preparations, I have ever tried, (and I have tried many) is in my Opinion the *common Vinum benedictum,* or Infusion of Glass of Antimony in Wine‖.—It is surprising we should seek for any other, as this possesses the whole Virtues of Antimony. You may make it a rough Emetic in a large Dose, you may give it in a few Drops, so as merely to excite perspiration:—With it you may puke, you may purge, you may sweat;—from ten to fifty, or sixty Drops it is an Attenuant, Altera-

* *Mart Rulandi Curat empiric. passim.*

†See *Memoires de l'Academie royale des Sciences, ann.* 1720.

‖ *Vid. Obs nostr. de Aere, &c. Vol. I. p.* 140. there called *Essentia Antimonii.*

tive, Diaphoretic and Diuretic; a few more gently purge; and every one knows a large Dose strongly vomits: What will any other Preparation of Antimony do more? Here it is in *solutis Principiis*, as the Chemists speak, in mere *Effluvia* as it were, in the most highly attenuated Manner, and most intimately and adequately mixed with the *Menstruum*; capable of passing and affecting the most intricate *Mœanders* of the very minutest Vessels, and yet powerful enough to stimulate the great alimentary Canal.—The common solid Preparations of Antimony are either a mere *inert Calx*, or very uncertain in their Operations, sometimes very rough, sometimes lying a long Time in the Stomach and Bowels, and exciting very untoward Symptoms; whereas this quickly acts, and as quickly passes off.—It certainly is an admirable Attenuant and Deobstruent, without heating a tenth Part so much as volatile alkalious Salts, and in most Cases much more safe and efficacious, particularly in the Disease now treated of.—In a Word it much more deserves the Name of a *Catholicon* than any of the boasted *Nostrums*, that are quacked upon the World by the great *W—d*, or the meanest Itinerant.—In good Hands it will certainly do great Things.—The timid, low, insipid Practice of some is almost as dangerous, as the bold unwarranted Empiricism of others; Time and Opportunity, never to be regained, are often lost by the former; whilst the latter, by a *bold Push*, sends you off the Stage in a Moment.

Blisters should never be neglected in a *Peripneumonia notha*, as not only serviceable from their attenuating and stimulating Quality, but also as they drain off Part of the Morbid Colluvies: A large one to the Neck should always be set on at the Begining, and Epispastics to the Legs and Thighs are often found to relieve the Head and Breast, when other Methods fail.—But as it frequently happens, in this Disorder, that the Limbs grow torpid and coldish, a very bad Symptom! they should be well rubbed before the Blisters are laid on, and then well wrapped up in Flannel (which by the Way is frequently also necessary in low nervous Fevers); for this very much promotes the Rising of the Blisters, and the consequent Discharge.

When comatose Symptoms and a very difficult Respiration remain after Bleeding, you may draw off more Blood by cupping and scarifying the Neck and Shoulders, when you cannot venture to open a Vein again; and this hath frequently a surprising good Effect: In a very threatening Case you should blister on the Scarifications.

Frequent Stools are certainly useful in this Disorder. *Sydenham* advises Purging every other Day* after bleeding once and again, but I think this is over-doing it in both Respects: For though Bleeding, and Purging too, may be necessary at the Begining; yet it is very seldom proper to repeat the former, and the latter must be managed with some Caution, especially when repeated. For the Patient is apt to fall into Faintness, cold Sweats, *&c.* unless properly supported during the Operation; which indeed may be easily done; but surely in most such Cases it requires more than Small-beer, and Water-gruel, to do it.—There is one Thing to be observed, as to both these Evacuations, and that is, that if the Sick spit largely a concocted Matter, which is sometimes the Case even in this Peripneumony, neither one nor the other is proper; and laxative Clysters or mild *Eccoprotics* only should be given, at least during the copious Expectoration: and thin Mustard-whey, *Hydromel*, or pectoral Decoction, with a small Quantity of soft white Wine in them, should be given frequently to promote it.—*Hippocrates*, in several Places, advises *Hydromel*, and sweet and watery Wine† in Pleurisies and Peripneumonies, to promote Spitting. Diuretics in this Case, if we are happy enough to succeed with them, are of very great Service, especially provided we can promote a *foul hypostatical Urine:* But the Truth is, in this Disorder, very little is to be depended on Urine, either as to *Crisis*, or *Prognostic*; only a thin, pale, or limpid Urine is universally bad in pulmonic Disorders.

Nitre, *Sperma ceti*, Cinnabar, Saffron, *Pulv. contrayerv.* Camphire, *Sp. vol. oleos. Lac. ammoniac.* and *Oxymel scilliticum*, Decoctions of Figs, Liquorice and Elecampane, are the most adapted Parts of the *Materia medica* in this Distemper. The *saline Draughts*, made with *Salt or Spirit of Harts-horn and Juice of Lemon or distilled Vinegar*, are exceeding useful; as they promote Expectoration greatly, relieve the Difficulty of breathing, and commonly operate by Sweat, or Urine.—But Opiates and oily mucilaginous Medicines are hurtful, and so are the highly stimulant and volatile if given too early, though they sometimes have a good Effect towards the End.—But the different Degrees of Heat, Fever, and Difficulty of breathing, the State of the Pulse, Blood, and other concomitant Symptoms, can only determine in what Manner, and to what Degree, very attenuating and warm Medicines, or those of a cooler Kind, may be made Use of.

**Cap. de Peripneum. notha.*

†Ο τνος γλυκυς καὶ ὑδαξὴς, *Lib. III. de Morb. Sect.* xxiv. *Ed. Lind.*

CHAP. IV.

Of Pleurisies.

A Violent Pain on either Side of the Breast, attended with an acute Fever, is commonly called a *Pleurisy*; and this whether it arises from an Inflammation of the *intercostal Muscles*, the *Periosteum* of the Ribs, or the *Pleura* itself; which last indeed, in Strictness of speaking, is only the true Pleurisy, the former being Species of an inflammatory Rheumatism, and are called *bastard*, or *spurious Pleurisies.*—However as they greatly affect the Respiration, when violent, they are always attended with much more ill Consequence than rheumatic Pains in other Parts of the Body, and demand a particular Regard, and a speedy Removal.

For as the Violence of the Pain hinders a due Expansion of the *Thorax*, the Respiration is immediately affected; hence, the Lungs not being sufficiently inflated, the Blood cannot pass freely from the pulmonic Arteries to the pulmonic Veins, and so into the left Ventricle of the Heart: Whence a Congestion, and some Degree of Stagnation of the Blood in the Lungs will arise.—Now as the right Ventricle of the Heart is continually throwing more Blood into the pulmonic Artery, its Branches become more and more distended, till at length they are rendered so very turgid, as to press on and obstruct the Branches also of the bronchial Arteries; and thus an Inflammation of the Lungs, or a compleat Peripneumony, is often the Consequence of a true, or bastard Pleurisy, especially when the Blood is very viscid.—Indeed whatever interrupts a free Inspiration and Expiration is apt to produce this.—Thus oftentimes a Quinsy brings on a Peripneumony, the free Passage of the Air, through the *Glottis* into the Lungs, being obstructed.—*Frederick Hoffman** takes Notice that even flatulent and spasmodic Colics, continuing any Time, are often succeeded by Pleurisies and Peripneumonies; the Pains, Spasms and Flatulence impeding the free Action of the Diaphragm;—and partly also, as he says, by hindering a due Passage of the Blood through the *Viscera of the Abdomen*, by which too much is thrown on the Lungs, Pleura, *&c.*—Very strait Lacing,

* *Consult. medicinal. Tom. I. Francos.* 1734. 4*to, p.* 450.

and Straining for a fine Shape, hath made many a fine Girl spit Blood, and ruined the Lungs, by preventing a full and easy Inspiration.—A fractured Rib, or even a simple Contusion of the Breast, very often brings on an *Hæmoptoe*, Cough, *&c.*—In Truth when any of the Muscles, that are but even subservient to Respiration, are greatly affected, peripneumonic Symptoms may come on. *Monsieur Mery** mentions the Case of a young Man, wounded in the Tendon of the *Pectoralis major*, who was forthwith seized with a very great Difficulty of breathing, and an acute Fever.—In a word all Kinds of Pains in the Breast, and Pleurisies especially, are in a peculiar Manner dangerous; as they are very apt to bring on more or less of a Peripneumony, by causing a great Interruption to regular and easy Respiration.—And this is the Reason, why we meet with many more pleuritic Fevers, accompanied with peripneumonic Symptoms, than true and exquisite Pleurisies: Where a severe Pain of the Breast is attended with an acute Fever, Load at Breast, Cough, difficulty of breathing, Expectoration, or Spiting of Blood; this is always the Case, and is very properly denominated a *Pleuroperipneumony.*—Indeed it sometimes happens, that, upon the coming on of the Peripneumony, the Pain of the Side ceases; which may happen, when the Infarction of the Lungs is so great, that little Blood passes from the right Ventricle of the Heart to the left, and the *Aorta* is not half supplied with Blood: So that the Powers of Nature sinking for Want of it, all tends to an universal Stagnation, and the Patients become as it were insensible, or, as *Aretæus*† says, complain of nothing, though their Pulse intermits, and their Extremities are cold. I have seen several such Instances.—About four Years since one *Mr. Cam,* a Sailor, was seized with a compleat *Paraplegia* about the 9th Day of a *Pleuroperipneumony*, and about twenty-four Hours before his Death.—It is a fatal Symptom therefore when the pleuritic Pain suddenly ceases, and yet the Difficulty of breathing and Load at Breast still continue, or encrease.—And the following *Aphorism* is most certainly true: "*A Peripneumony supervening a Pleurisy is dangerous*‖."

But the Nature and Consequences of Pleurisies will more fully appear from the following Considerations.

1st. The inflamed *Pleura* is apt to cleave to the external Mem-

**Mémoires de l'Académie royale des Sciences,* 1713.
†*De Pulmonaria.*
‖*Hipp. Aphorism.* II. *Sect.* vii.

brane of the Lungs, and propagate the Inflammation to them; and this will more easily happen, when either by Nature, or Disease, a previous Cohesion had been partly formed: Hence those, that have once laboured under a Pleuro-peripneumony, are often afterwards subject to the like Disorder; the *Callosity*, as I may call it, formed by the *Concretion*, straitening the Blood-vessels of the *Pleura*, and making them more liable to be obstructed by a fizy Blood for the future.—Not to mention the more or less Impediment, which the Adhesion of the Lungs to the Pleura gives to full and free Respiration.

2dly. As the external Membrane of the Lungs is only a Continuation of the *Pleura* itself, the Inflammation may be diffused from one Part of the *Pleura* to another, and even to that which immediately invests the Lungs; for it may spread a considerable Space, just as we often see a small inflammatory Speck on the Eye soon spread into a general Inflammation of the whole Globe, Eye-lids, *&c.*—Besides the Inflammation may primarily fall on this Membrane of the Lungs, and then Pains, altogether like the pleuritic, will arise, though the internal Membrane of the *Thorax* (or Pleura) may not be affected.—I am quite of the experienced *Hoffman's** Opinion, that this is often the Case.

3dly. The very *Mediastinum* is but a *Duplicature* of the *Pleura*, and an Inflammation may attack any Part of it, or be propagated to it; in which Case very acute Pains are felt under the *Sternum*, or between the Shoulder-blades; This we sometimes meet with, and it is generally attended with great Danger.—Both *Hippocrates*† and *Aretæus*‖ take Notice of a *dorsal Pleurisy*, in which the Pain shoots from the Spine to the Breast-bone, attended with an *Orthopnœa*, Cough, and a very difficult and small Expectoration.—This seems to be the Case mentioned.—Sometimes the Pain is forward and directly under the *Sternum*, where the *Mediastinum* is attached to it, and in Consequence of it Apostems have been found in that Part.—When the Pain seems to lie very deep in the Chest, with a great Load and Anxiety, Palpitation of the Heart, and a constant Inclination as it were to raise a Cough, the *Pericardium* (the external Membrane of which is also from the *Pleura*) is commonly inflamed.—Where the Pain is spread all over the Breast, with a great

* *Cap. de Febribus pneumonicis, Tom. IV. Parte* i.

† *Lib. III. de Morbis, Sect.* xxi. *Edit. Lindeni.*

‖ *Cap. de Pleuritide.*

Oppression, and perpetual darting pricking Pains here and there; not only the *Mediastinum*, but the external Membrane of both Lobes of the Lungs seems to be inflamed: The great Difficulty of Breath, Load, and Anxiety, perpetual Cough, and constant Desire of sitting up erect, shew this to be the Case; and a very dangerous one it is, as well as an Inflammation of the *Pericardium.*—Inflammations of the *Mediastinum*, *Pericardium*, and Membranes of the Lungs, seem to be what the Ancients called an *Erysipelas of the Lungs; Hippocrates* describes it as an acute Fever, with great Pain in the fore Parts of the Breast and in the Back, with much Load, seeming Fulness, and a dry Cough*.

4thly. The upper Membrane of the *Diaphragm* is likewise from the *Pleura*, and may be either primarily inflamed, or secondarily from the Inflammation of the Pleura: And this certainly happens more commonly than is imagined.—This is called a *Paraphrenitis*, and is attended with a very acute Fever, and a very violent Pain extended from the lower Ribs to the lowest *Vertebræ* of the Back, a short, convulsive, *singultose* Kind of breathing, a vast Anxiety and Uneasiness, dry Cough, Hiccup and Delirium; an excessive Pain is particularly felt on every Inspiration, which darts itself from the Pit of the Stomach to the very Loins; the *Hypochondrium* of the Side affected is drawn inwards, and upwards† under the Ribs, and the Abdomen is scarce perceptibly moved in Respiration, but remains fixed and convulsed as it were by the Violence of the Pain, in attempting an inspiration.

Any Part therefore of this widely expanded Membrane being inflamed, a Kind of Pleurisy is generated, in which the Lungs themselves by *Continuity*, *Contiguity, Cohesion*, or *Sympathy*, will soon become greatly affected.—Nay, the Lungs may, and often are found to adhere to the *Mediastinum* and *Diaphragm*, as well as to the *Pleura* commonly so called.—But if the Lungs should not adhere to any Part of the *Pleura*, peripneumonic Symptoms may supervene an Inflammation of it; because the Let and Hinderance it gives to a regular Respiration will greatly interrupt a due Circulation of the Blood through the Lungs.—The same may be said with Respect to any considerable inflammation of the intercostal Muscles, or *Periosteum* of the Ribs.—Indeed in these Cases the peripneumonic

* *Lib. I. de Morbis, Sect.* xiii. *Edit. Linden.*

† *Si septum transversum percussum, est, præcordia sursum contrahuntur. Celsus, Lib. V. Cap.* xxvi.

Symptoms may not presently come on, nor commonly do they till after two, three, or four Days; but as the inflammatory Pain hinders a due Expansion of the *Thorax*, and a sufficient *Inflation of the Lungs*, they at length also may become greatly affected.

These then being too often the Consequences of pleuritic Fevers, we should endeavour to take off the Inflammation in a true, or bastard Pleurisy, as soon as possible, by large and repeated Bleeding, cooling nitrous Medicines and Drinks, Fomentations, Opiates, *&c.*—In a Word, we should treat the Case as a *mere Inflammation of the Membranes, Muscles, or Periosteum*; but when a Load at Breast, Cough, Expectoration, *&c.* come on, we must have a Regard to these also, as well as to the Pain of the Side, *&c.*

And it is that the Nature, Situation, and Difference of the Diseases of the Breast, and Lungs, may be more easily known and distinguished in Practice, that I have been so particular in describing them: For it would be no small Absurdity to give Expectorants, *oleaginous Linctus*, and Pectorals, in a simple Inflammation of the Muscles of the Breast, or Pleura; even although a slight symptomatic Cough, and some Difficulty of breathing should attend, especially at the very Access of the Fever; whereas well timed Bleeding, and a proper Regimen would have soon carried off the Disorder.—On the other Hand, it would be altogether as wrong to rest solely on Bleeding and Fomentations, where the Lungs also were primarily, or even secondarily, affected in any considerable Degree.

The Distinction of Pleurisies into *true* and *bastard* hath a real Foundation in Nature, and is of some Import in Practice; for when the intercostal Muscles only are inflamed, much more is to be expected from topical Applications, as Fotus, Cataplasms, Blisters, Cupping, and the like, than when the Pain of the Side is from an Inflammation of the *Pleura*, or external Membrane of the Lungs.—The Soreness to the Touch, the Pain on lying on the affected Side, and chiefly on a full Inspiration, the Tumor and Redness of the Part which sometimes appear, distinguish this from the internal Pleurisy.

Besides there are some Pains of the Side, and those too pretty severe, which arise from a sharp acrid Defluxion on the Muscles of the Breast, and Periosteum of the Ribs; and which much sooner give Way to topical Applications, edulcorant Medicines, and proper Purges, than to Bleeding, which in such Cases is no further necessary, than to take off a *Plethora*, if it subsists.—Indeed where an acrimonious Humor is the Causes, you may bleed and bleed on to very little Purpose, but that of weakening your Patient.—Will Bleeding cure obstinate scorbutic or venereal Pains? It may as well remove the Pain from a rotten Tooth, or a Thorn in the Flesh.

The Ancients well distinguished between wandering rheumatic, or flatulent Pains about the Breast and Side, and the truly pleuritic. *Hippocrates* justly styles them, Ἀλγήματα ἰσχνῶς ἑστηκότα ἄσημα *, and forbids Bleeding in them: These they attempted to cure by Fomentations, Purging, *&c.* not by Bleeding; whereas the fixed, *systrophic* Inflammation of the Breast, as the *Commentators call it*, always required Bleeding.—And we eventually find erratic, scorbutic, rheumatic Pains much better carried off by Purging, Fotus, Diaphoretics and Edulcorants, than by Bleeding.—Some of them indeed give Way to nothing but Mercurials, Antimonials, anodyne Plasters, Cupping, or Blistering; and some wear off only by Time, Patience, and Exercise. When the Pains are at the Bottom of the Thorax, in the *Hypochondria*, or below the Midriff, attended with *Borborygmi*, and a tumid Abdomen; Clystering, or Purging, is unquestionably proper: And yet these Pains are sometimes very acute, and, from the Inflation of the Intestines by Wind, oftentimes accompanied with no small Difficulty of breathing; but as *Aretæus* observes, they are very improperly called *pleuritic.*—I have many Timesseen such Complaints vanish immediately on the Use of a Clyster, or a few Stools, to the Surprise of those, who were ignorant of the Cause.—Bleeding in this Case always encreases the Flatulence and Pain.—This is entirely consonant to the *Hippocratic* Doctrine, and the Truth of Things; for the great Dictator of Physic says expressly, when the Pain is below the *Septum transversum*, and the Abdomen is tumid, you should purge gently with black Hellebore, *Peplium*, *Silphium*, to which add Cummin, Anise, *&c.* that it may carry off the Wind as well as the Stool †.

But in all these Cases the Pulse, Degree of Fever, the Tongue, Situation of the Pain, and Manner of Breathing, pretty clearly discover to the judicious Practitioner what is the Matter, and what is to be done.—When the Pain of the Thorax is violent, the Pulse hard, tense, and quick, the Fever high; the Pains may be pro-

* Shifting, erratic, slight Pains, *without the true pleuritic Symptoms; Coac. Prænot.* 491. *Edit. Foësii.*—Compare this with the Caution about Bleeding at the End of *Duretus*'s second Book on the *Coac. Prænot.*

† *De Victu acutor. Sect.* xiii. *Edit. Lindeni.*

nounced pleuritic, especially when a *Rigor* preceded.—True pleuritic Disorders almost always begin with a *Rigor*, and the Pulse is very hard and tense, like the Vibrations of a *Cord*: The Pains are very sharp, pricking, and fixed, not tensive and shifting, as the flatulent; nor uncertain, wide and wandering, as the rheumatic.—The Hardness of the Pulse is one of the most *pathognomonic* Signs of an Inflammation of membranous Parts; when therefore Pains lie under the *Sternum*, or shoot from the Spine to the Breast-bone, you may guess the *Mediastinum* is inflamed, by the Tension of the Pulse.—The Lungs, as *Aretæus** says, being insensible (at least much less sensible) a *Vomica* is often formed in the Lungs without much attendant Pain. The *Membranes* of any *Organ* are vastly more sensible than what is called its *Parenchyma*, the Ureters than the Kidnies, the Membranes of the Brain than the Brain.—The Hardness of the Pulse then, and Violence of the Pain, may be the chief *Diagnostics* in Disorders of the Thorax, and greatly determine as to Bleeding, *&c.*—I think the Situation of the Pain is not so much to be regarded, as some make it; for as any part of the Pleura, intercostal Muscles, or Periosteum of the Ribs may be inflamed; the Pain may be felt in any Part of the Thorax: And I have known as severe Pains near the bastard Ribs, as in any other part. *Hippocrates* and his Commentators determine Bleeding to be then peculiarly proper, when the Pain shoots up to the Clavicle and Shoulder; but in my Opinion, when the Pain is very severe in any other Part, it is equally necessary:—The Pain is very low in a *Paraphrenitis*, and yet none more loudly demands it. When the *Pectoralis major* and *Serratus anticus minor* are inflamed, the Pain cannot but dart up to the Shoulder, as their *Tendons* are inserted near its *Articulation*: This is often the Case in a bastard Pleurisy, and is most effectually relieved by Bleeding and Formentations; but these would be as necessary, if the intercostal Muscles, or Periosteum of any of the Ribs, were inflamed.

Though some Pains of the Side may be greatly different from the pleuritic, and require much less Bleeding; they should never be neglected, especially if they considerably obstruct the Respiration: For then they are always followed with very ill Consequences; a strong Instance of which you have in the following History.

About *Christmas* 1728. Mr. *T—ll*, a worthy sober Gentleman, about thirty, of a thin Habit of Body, but a lively active Disposition,

**Cap. de Pulmonar.*

was seized with a Pain in his *right Side*, and grew a little feverish; the Pain was so slight that he never confined himself. He was bled however, and took some few Things from his Surgeon.—But finding the Pain of his Side daily encreasing, about three Weeks, or a Month, after the first Attack, he consulted me.—I found him under hectical Heats, a short Cough and Difficulty of breathing, which last he said proceeded merely from the Pain of his side: He expectorated little, and that with Difficulty; and it was now sometimes slightly tinged with Blood.—I ordered him to be bled, to take an oily expectorating Mixture, *Lac ammoniac. Oxymel. scillitic.* the saline Draughts and pectoral Decoction, and kept him to a cool diluting Regimen. By these Means in a very few Days he began to spit off a vast quantity of purulent, bloody, and foetid Matter, which proceeded from a *Vomica* in the *left Lobe* of the Lungs; for he felt a Soreness in, and said that the Matter came from, a *Place* to the *left* of the *Sternum*, towards the Bottom of the *Thorax.*—At length very little was expectorated, and that neither fœtid, nor bloody; and his Cough daily abated, nor did any great Load at his Breast remain: A pectoral balsamic Decoction of the *Bark* soon also took off his remaining Heats and Sweats; so that I flattered myself with Hopes of his speedy Recovery.—But, notwithstanding all these promising Symptoms, the Pain of his *right Side* still continued, exactly in the same Place where it first began; nay it soon became exceeding violent, so that I thought it necessary to bleed him again, and even repeat it; I ordered also emollient Fomentations, and an anodyne Plaster of *Opium, Camphire*, and *Emplastr. è Cymino*; and, these not availing, cupping on the Part with Scarifications.—All was in vain, for the Pain daily encreased, and nothing gave the least Ease, or Sleep, but repeated Opiates.—At last the Part began to swell considerably, and manifest Signs of an *Abscess* came on, which I endeavoured by all proper Methods to promote.—In a few Days the Surgeon opened it, from whence issued an immense Quantity of purulent Matter, so much, that we imagined it came partly from the *Cavity of the Thorax.*—Upon further Examination we found two of the Ribs foul and black, and two Penetrations, one between the fifth and sixth of the true Ribs (which were *carious*) and the other between the fourth and fifth, reckoning downwards. He, being exceeding weak, hectical and emaciated, died *March* 29th, 1729.

On examining the Body some of the intercostal Muscles, Part of the *Serratus anticus major*, and the supreme Portion of the *Obliquus descendens* appeared *black* and *sphacelated*, and the Impostume had extended itself almost home to the *Spine* of the *Back*: The lower Part of the *Pleura* was quite black, and the *Diaphragm also on that Side, livid.* The *upper Perforation* entered the *right Lobe* of the Lungs, which, for a considerable Way round it, was purulent.—In the left Lobe we observed a Kind of *Callosity*, of a pretty large Extent, where probably the *Vomica* lay; and near the *Vertebræ* a large *Tumor*, bigger than a Turkey-egg, in a State of Suppuration: There were several other small Tubercles, some very hard and almost stony; some suppurated and full of *Pus.*—Both Lobes of the Lungs were greatly diseased, and, in some Places, quite livid.—They adhered firmly to the *Pleura* in a vast many Places, some of the Adhesions of a pretty large Extent, some by a Sort of fibrous Ligaments.—In the *right Cavity of the Thorax* was about half a Pint of very fœtid dark-coloured Matter.

Probably some Obstructions were formed in this Gentleman's Lungs antecedent to the Pain of his Side, as he had been sometimes subject to a short dry Cough; but I am persuaded the sharp Humor, that fell on the Ribs and intercostal Muscles, by hindering a free Respiration, greatly contributed towards the Obstructions and Suppurations in his Lungs; and by preventing also a due Expansion of the *Thorax*, it might encrease, at least, the Adhesion of the Lungs to the Pleura.

I shall conclude this Chapter with a Word or two on the Method of treating inflammatory Pleurisies:—In which, without all Doubt, drawing off more or less Blood is indispensably necessary, previous to any other Attempt of Relief: The Strength of the Patient, Pulse and Fever, the Violence of the Pain and Difficulty of breathing must determine the Quantity.—But let me add, the Quality of the Blood should also be nicely inspected; for a dense sizy Blood not only indicates an abundant Quantity of the red Globules, but likewise its inflammatory Disposition, and that the Patient, if Need be, can well bear large and repeated Bleeding.

It should be duly considered, that if an Inflammation of the *Pleura, &c.* is not timely abated by Bleeding, or resolved by proper diluting, antiphlogistic, emollient Drinks and Medicines; it cannot but end in an Impostumation, or Gangrene. Besides these Pleurisies rarely fail of bringing on peripneumonic Symptoms, if of any Continuance; and therefore we cannot be too early and earnest in endeavouring to take off the Inflammation: For the Pain thence arising greatly embarrasses the Respiration, and of Course the due Circulation of the Blood through the Lungs; which being now also in a very viscid State (the immediate Occasion of the original pleuritic Inflammation) is much more apt to stick in the ultimate Branches of the pulmonic, or bronchial Arteries, than if it was more thin and fluxile. This is the Reason, why Pains of the Side, from Inflammation, bring on Peripneumonies much more frequently, than when from a mere acrimonious Defluxion, or the like.—Here therefore *Celsus*'s Maxim is certainly right, *Remedium . . . est magni & recentis doloris, sanguis missus*; and what he had is true likewise, *at si . . . vetustior casus est, . . . serum id auxilium est**.

An emollient cooling Clyster should immediately succeed Bleeding, especially if the Body is costive, which not only empties the Intestines of gross Excrements and *Flatus*, but also derives a greater Quantity of Blood through the descending *Aorta* and *Iliacs*, and in both Respects eases the superior Parts.† *Hippocrates* constantly advises to clyster in the Begining of Pleurisies, and gives this exceeding good Caution: That we should neither suffer the Body to be too costive, lest it encrease the Fever, nor too loose, lest both the Strength and Spitting fail‖.

This done let the pained Part be fomented with a Decoction of *Sem. Lini.—Fœnugræc. Flor Chamæm.* In Milk and Water.—This was also the Practice of the Ancients; *Hippocrates*§ says Fomentations should be tried both at the very Begining, and afterwards, to resolve the pleuritic Pains: These, both of the dry and humid Kind, he constantly advises in Pleurisies.—I have often seen them succeed, when repeated Bleeding had proved ineffectual.—Pain, especially inflammatory Pain, always arises from too great a Tension of the Fibres which emollient Fomentations, by relaxing, take off. I greatly prefer humid Fomentations, or Cataplasms, to any Thing of a dry Heat in an inflammatory Pain of the Breast, or Side, as they without all Doubt much more efficaciously relax: *Hippocrates* himself advises against using the *dry Stupes*** too long, and recommends those that are moist‡ near the *Crisis.—Celsus* says, we should use the dry and hot, when the Inflammation is a little abated, and then

* *Lib. IV. Cap.* vi.

† *De Victu acutor. Sect.* lii.

‖ *Lib. III. de Morbis, Sect.* xvii.

§ *De Vict. acut. Sect.* xi, xii. *Edit. Linden.*

** *Ibid. Sect.* xii.

‡ *Lib. III. de Morbis, Sect.* xxiii.

pass on to the *Malagmata**. I commonly apply an anodyne Plaster of *Opium* ℥i, *Camphire* ℈i, *Emplastr. è Cymino*, after due Fomentations, with very good Success, but always first try the humid Fotus.—In very threatening Circumstances, Fomentations also may be applied to the Abdomen, *Inguina, &c.* which, by taking down the too great Stricture of the Fibres in general, will lessen the Impetuosity of the Blood.—Emollient *Baths* would be more effectual, when they can be conveniently used; *Hippocrates* says they relieve Pains of the Back, Sides, and Breast: Their exceeding good Effects in *Colics, and nephritic Paroxysms*, should prompt us to try them in very violent obstinate Pleurisies, and a *Paraphrenitis*. —The Ancients supposed that warm Applications digested the Matter, and promoted Expectoration; the latter they certainly do by easing the Pain, and giving more Liberty to the intercostal Muscles, *&c.* to expand and contract the Thorax, and pump up the Matter; hence in *Pleuro-pneumonies* they cannot but be of very considerable Service, even in that Respect.

Nitrous Medicines, with a cooling, emollient, diluting Regimen, should be forthwith entered upon. Thin Whey, a Decoction of Barley and red Poppies, Emulsions, and such like, answer all the Intentions of Drink; and Nitre both cools and attenuates the Blood: With these should be joined gentle Anodynes, repeated as there may be Occasion; *Elixir paregoricum* and *Diacodium* seem to me the most adapted: To these may be added *Sperma ceti*, a soft relaxing animal Oil, very penetrating, though not heating; and, where the Rigidity of the Fibres is very great, the cool vegetable Oils, as of Linseed, or Almonds, may be given with Advantage. That an emollient relaxing Method is indicated, in the Cure of Pleurisies, is evident from hence, *viz.* That the strong and laborious Persons of very rigid Fibres, and dry Constitutions, are most subject to this Disease, and suffer most from it, and withal that it rages most in cold and dry Seasons.

The Violence of Pain unquestionably demands the Use of Opiates, after Bleeding, which prudently interposed are certainly of exceeding great Service.—As Pain is a *Stimulus*, which greatly quickens the Circulation, and heats the Blood, and derives likewise more than natural to the pained Part; it cannot but encrease the Inflammation—A Thorn in the Flesh will cause some Degree of Fever, and an Inflammation around it.—Moreover when a sharp

* *Lib. IV. Cap.* 6.

Cough attends, as in Pleuro-peripneumonies, it should be mitigated by *Diacodium,* or the like; else the great Agitation, it causes, will also encrease the Inflammation.—It is true indeed, these demand some Degree of Caution and Prudence in the Use of them; therefore ever remember, before you enter upon them, the Lancet is not to be sparingly used, when the Pain is very violent, the Pulse very hard, quick and tense, and the Fever high.—The following Instance shews what may, and must be done sometimes in Pleurisies and *Pleuro-pneumonies,* when the Attack is with extreme violence.

About four Years since a strong plethoric Gentleman, about forty, was seized with a Fever and a violent Pain of his Side: He was immediately bled to sixteen or eighteen Ounces:—This abated the Pain.—He got up, sat by the Fire in a smoaky Chamber, drank near a Quart of cold Cyder, fell into a vast Rigor, succeeded by a high Fever, excessive Pain of his Side and Breast, great Difficulty of breathing, Delirium, and the most incessant terrible Cough I ever heard, which pumped up great Quantities of fresh frothy Blood.—I was obliged to bleed him three Times in twenty-four Hours, and to give him *seven Grains of solid Laudanum, besides two or three Ounces of Diacodium,* in that short Space of Time;—and this, and this only (for he would take no other Medicine) happily recovered him.—This indeed is a very extraordinary Instance:—But the Method, which is above recommended, I have in a Multitude of Cases experienced to be very safe and very effectual; infinitely more so, I think, than the *Sanguis hirci, Priapus tauri,* and the other Whimsies which *Helmont,* so greatly extolls in appeasing the *Archæus,* and quieting the *Pleura furens**; notwithstanding he is so very arch and severe on the Sons of *Galen* and the *Schools,* for attempting to cure Pleurisies by Bleeding.

In several epidemic Pleurisies, I have known easy Sweating, especially after the third or fourth Day, of very great Advantage; and, with this View, have often added Camphire to the Nitre, *&c.* which, joined with small Doses of *Elixir paregoricum* out of thin warm Whey, or Ptisan, seldom or never fails of answering the Intention.—In chilly wet Seasons, and Persons formerly subject to catarrhal, or cold rheumatic Disorders, this is a very proper Method, when a due Quantity of Blood hath been previously drawn off: In such Cases also gentle Purging is useful.—It is certain, from the best Observations, that in some Constitutions of the Air

* *Vid.* Helmont. *Pleura furens.*

Patients, under pleuritic Diseases, will not bear the Loss of much Blood, particularly in continued wet foggy Weather: In general, we find they sustain the Loss with much better Effect, and less Inconveniency, in a cold dry Spring than in a wet Summer, or a rainy Autumn. Nay, there are some Pleurisies, at least vulgarly so called, that will admit of little or no Bleeding, in which the Pain of the Side seems a mere Symptom, not the Disease; as the Pains and Soreness preceding, or attending putrid malignant Fevers, Small-pox, *&c.* are not properly rheumatic, but purely symptomatical.—Such Pains then arise from Acrimony, not Inflammation, and are to be cured by Diluents, Diaphoretics, Eccoprotics, Blistering, *&c.* not by Bleeding, which is forbidden by the Ancients where *Bile* (by which they meant Acrimony) is greatly predominant.

It was an Observation of *Asclepiades**, that the People of *Rome* and *Athens* did not bear Bleeding in Pleurisies and Peripneumonies as well as those about the *Hellespont*; the former lying to the South, and in a much more warm and moist Air than the latter, who were much exposed to cold dry northerly and easterly Winds: *Hollerius* makes the same Observation with Respect to the People of *Paris*, who lie pretty cold, and the Inhabitants of the southern Parts of *France*, who are more to the South and much warmer†.—Indeed, within a much narrower Compass, I have once and again taken Notice, that an epidemic Disorder, which in low warm Places near the Sea proved only a slightly catarrhal Fever, and scarce required any Manner of Bleeding, hath, in the neighbouring cold and high Exposures, been attended with severe pleuro-peripneumonic Symptoms, and demanded no small Evacuation of Blood.—Without all Doubt, the very Constitution of the Solids and Fluids differs considerably, according to the different Situation of the Inhabitants.—Upon the whole then let me add this *Corollary*, that in Practice we not only ought to consider the peculiar Nature of the Epidemic, but also of the Season, and the Constitution of the Patients.

* *Vid. Cæl. Aurelian. Lib. II. Cap.* xxii. *de Morbis acutis & chronicis, Amst.* 1722. 4*to.*

† *Holler. in Aphorism* 2. *Hippocr. Sect.* i.

A P P E N D I X.

A Method for preserving the Health of Seamen in long Cruises and Voyages.

IT is well known what vast Numbers of Sailors we have lost within these few Years, by terrible scorbutic Disorders, owing chiefly to bad Provisions, bad Water, bad Beer, *&c.* the unavoidable Consequence of long Cruises and Voyages: For the Provisions will naturally decay, the best Beef and Pork corrupt, the Water spoil, and the Beer (at least such as the Navy is supplied with) will not keep good very long. Of Course, the long and constant Use of such Provisions must by Degrees taint the Juices of the Body, produce great Acrimony in the Blood, and dispose it daily more and more to a State of Putrefaction. These Effects will be considerably augmented by living continually in a moist, salt Atmosphere, and breathing the foul, polluted Air between Decks. Constant Experience shews this to be the Case. I have known more than a thousand Men put ashore sick out of one single Squadron, after a three Months Cruise, most of them highly scorbutic; besides many that died in the Voyage. The Fleet returns to its Port; fresh Air, wholesome Liquor, fresh Provisions, especially proper Fruits and Herbage, soon purify the Blood and Juices of the Sick, and restore their Health. The fresh Air, Provisions, Fruits, and Garden-stuff, which the *English* and *Dutch* meet with at *St. Helena*, and the *Cape of Good Hope*, are of the highest Advantage to them in their *East-India* Voyages; without which they always become extreamly sickly.

Physicians well know, that the most effectual Method of correcting an alcalescent Acrimony of the Blood, and of preventing the further Advances of Putrefaction in the Humors, is by vegetable and mineral Acids; the former of which are much the safest, and may be given in Draughts, the other only by Drops.

That the State of the Blood, in the common Sea-scurvy, is of this

Nature, appears from the stinking Breath of the Sick, their rotten corroded Gums, high-coloured fœtid Urine, sordid Ulcers, black, blue and brown Spots, and Eruptions on the Skin, frequent feverish Heats, foul Tongues, bilious and bloody Dysenteries, which more or less always attended it. Now it is also well known, that a vegetable acescent Diet and Regimen, fresh Air, fresh Provisions, subacid and vinous Drinks, are its certain and speedy Cure, when not very far advanced. Apples, Oranges, and Lemons, alone, have been often known to do surprising Things in the Cure of very deplorable scorbutic Cases, that arose from bad Provisions, bad Water, *&c.* in long Voyages.

But what will cure will prevent. If therefore such a Diet and Regimen can be used at Sea, it will prove a Kind of a continual Antidote to the rank putrescent Qualities of the common Ships Provision, and correct, at least very much lessen, the ill Effects. And it is eventually found, that the Officers, who carry Wine, Cyder, Lemons, fresh Provisions, *&c.* are infinitely less affected with the Scurvy, than the poor common Sailors, who are not so provided.

Is it practicable then to introduce such a general Regimen into the Navy? I think it is; and, from Reason and Experience, I recommend the following Method.

Let all Ships, that are to proceed on a long Cruise or Voyage, be supplied with a sufficient Quantity of sound, generous Cyder; the rougher, provided it is perfectly sound, the better. If apples are found of such vast Service in the Scurvy, surely the Juice of them, when become a vinous Liquor, cannot but be very salutary; and seems exceedingly well adapted, as a common Drink, to correct by its Acidity the alcalescent putrefying Quality of bad, corrupt Provisions. This Cyder should be at least three Months old before it is served in, and quite fine. If it be too new, and foul, it is apt to give severe Colics: It should be racked off once at least from its gross Ley into good and sweet Vessels, which will contribute to its becoming fine, and prevent it from growing ropy, in which State it is good for nothing. But if some of it should turn to Vinegar, which may frequently happen, it will still be very serviceable; but it is found, when well managed, to keep good and sound even to the *Indies.*

Every Sailor should have at least a Pint of Cyder a Day, besides Beer and Water. And I would advise also a frequent and free Use of Vinegar in the Seamen's Diet; especially when the Provisions begin to grow rancid. Besides this, the Decks, *&c.* should be frequently washed or sprinkled with Vinegar; after having drawn the gross and foul Air out of the Ship by Mr. *Sutton*'s Contrivance, or by Dr. *Hales*'s Ventilators; which should be done once at least every Day.

In autumnal Cruises a Quantity of Apples might be also carried, which, when well chosen and well put up in dry tight Casks, will keep very good for two or three Months. Even Lemons and Oranges wrapt in Flannel (or something that will imbibe their exhaling Moisture) kept in close dry Vessels, and pretty cool, may be preserved a long while also. If this is not so feasible, a Mixture of Lemon Juice and Rum (Shrub as they call it) may be carried in any Quantity; as it will keep a long Time, and would prove infinitely more wholesome than the nasty fiery poisonous Spirits, which are dealt about so largely in the Navy and elsewhere. By the bye, nothing would more effectually correct the pernicious Qualities of these Spirits than Lemon Juice.

In the Case of stinking Water, Juice of Lemon, Elixir of Vitriol, or Vinegar, should be always mixed with it, which will render it much less unwholesome: The *Roman* Soldiers drank *Posca* (*viz.* Water and Vinegar) for their common Drink, and found it very healthy and useful.

Elixir of Vitriol and Vinegar are already allowed to the Navy in large Quantities, and have been found greatly serviceable. And there was lately an Order issued for supplying the Ships of War with Cyder also, which I am morally certain will be of the highest Advantage, if properly and honestly managed. Indeed it hath already been actually found so in some few Men of War, and other Ships, where it hath been tried, even though in small Quantities. Let me add, that the Prize Wines, which are commonly low and thin, and very frequently spoil by keeping, might be distributed amongst the Sailors (especially in Want of Cyder) to very good Purpose.

This indeed may be deemed a very expensive Project; but, where the Lives of so many brave and useful People are in the Case, I think the Cost should by no Means come into Competition with the Advantage that may be received from it: The *Romans* constantly carried with them Vinegar and Wine in their Fleets and Armies, and the common Soldier and Sailor daily partook of both: Nay, they were at many other considerable Expences to preserve the Health of their Armies, *&c.* Now, if that glorious prudent People thought the Life of a *Roman* Soldier so valuable, and were at such Expence to preserve it; why should not we have as much Regard to that of a *British* Sailor, who is altogether as brave and as useful to the Commonwealth?

I cannot conclude without taking Notice, that the useful Method of impressing Seamen on their Return from long and tedious Voyages, void of Necessaries, chagrined at not seeing their Friends and Families, and most commonly in a bad Sate of Health, and not allowed Time and Opportunity to recover it, hath been the Bane of Thousands: And I could wish, for the Honour of the Nation, a Method of manning our Fleet could be found out more consistent with common Humanity and *British* Liberty.

Plymouth, Sept. 30, 1747.

A
DISSERTATION
ON THE
Malignant Ulcerous SORE-THROAT.

SINCE the Publication of my *Essay on Fevers*, I have had frequent Opportunities of making Observations on a Disease of the putrid, malignant Kind, which abundantly confirm my Notions of the Cause and Cure of Malignant pestilential Fevers.—I mean what is called the *Angina maligna*, or *Ulcerous Sore-Throat*, which hath appeared up and down this Kingdom for several Years, in some Places very common and exceedingly fatal, especially to Children.

The first accurate Account we had of this Distemper in *England*, was from the very ingenious Dr. *Fothergill*, in 1748.—But several of the *Spanish* and *Italian Physicians* have described exactly such a Kind of Disease, as raging with great Violence and Mortality in *Spain*, and several Parts of *Italy*, in the Begining of the last Century.—Perhaps the *Syrian* and *Ægyptian Ulcers* mentioned by *Aretæus Cappadox*, and the *pestilent ulcerated Tonsils*, we read of in *Ætius Amidenus*, were of this Nature;— and truly some of the Scarlet Fevers, mentioned by *Morton*, seem not much unlike it.

It is not above six, or seven Years since I met with it in this Town and Neighbourhood, though it raged with great Fatality in and about *Lostwithiel, St. Austle, Fowye*, and *Liskeard*, a Year or two before.—From the latter Part of the Year 1751 to *May* 1753 it was very common in this Town, and Places adjacent, especially in the Year 1752, and not only carried off Children, but several Adults.

As a faithful and accurate History of Diseases, their various Symptoms, and Methods of Cure, is the most effectual Way of promoting the Art of Healing, Physicians should describe with the utmost Care the Diseases they would treat of, and the good and bad Effects of any Method, or Medicines, they have used to remove them.—But in a more particular Manner is this necessary when any new, or uncommon Distemper occurs, of which the peculiar pathognomonic and diagnostic Signs should be carefully laid down, and a particular Account given of what Evacuations, Regimen, and Medicines were useful, or hurtful, in it.—And this Method I shall endeavour to pursue with the utmost Attention in the following Account.

A vast Quantity of Rain fell during the Year 1751, the Summer particularly was, in general, uncommonly wet, cold and frequently stormy.—At the Begining of *June* however we had exceeding hot Weather, and some very sultry Days also in *July* and *August*; the Atmosphere was almost always thick and moist, but the Barometer low commonly.—The Fruits of the Earth were crude, watery, and insipid; the Harvest was excessively bad, and the Grain of all Kinds suffered greatly.—Notwithstanding this we had but little Sickness, at least no very epidemical Distemper: But the Small-pox (brought in by *Conway*'s *Regiment*, in *May*) spread in this Town considerably in *July* and *August*; and there were then several putrid and miliary Fevers, in the southern Parts of this County.—Indeed, though we were not here very sickly, yet hypochondriacal and hysteric Disorders greatly prevailed, and there was a Kind of universal Inactivity and Lowness of Spirits every-where.

The Small-pox became much more common in the Autumn, and of a much worse Kind than they were at their first Appearance, and about the Mid-winter were very epidemic and fatal.—In the mean Time there were Abundance of Catarrhs, mucous and inflammatory Sore-Throats, some Pleurisies and Peripneumonies; and commonly Eruptions of the erysipelatous, or pustular Kind, attended all these Disorders.

The Weather still continued wet, and often very boisterous, the Wind various.—*December* was a cold Month, but wet from the 15th to the 25th.—The same Diseases continued, and about the End of the Year were several malignant ulcerous Sore-Throats up and down.

The Year 1752 began cold, wet, and frequently stormy, the Wind most commonly from the East, verging however considerably, now to the North, now to the South; the Barometer often very low, though at the Begining of *January* very high, with sharp Frost.—The Small-pox continued epidemic, often crude, crystalline, and undigested to the very End, sometimes very confluent, small and sessile; some black and bloody, and now and then attended with Petechiæ.—Pleuroperipneumonies, and Rheumatisms, were not uncommon: catarrhal and mucous Squinzies with much Cough, and a large thin Spitting, were very rife; and now also there were several malignant dangerous Sore-Throats with no small Degree of Fever.

Both at the Begining, and End, of *February*, the Mercury was high, and the Air clear, dry, and frosty; but, from the 8th to the 21st, there was much Rain with the Wind generally at South.—Many Small-pox were in the Town, though few in the Neighbourhood; several Pleurisies, Peripneumonies, and Rheumatisms, a vast Quantity of catarrhal, mucous Sore-Throats, and many inflammatory Squinzies; and still some of the malignant Kind.

The Weather was pretty cold and dry in *March*, especially at the Begining, and latter End; and the Barometer high, at no Time very low.—The Small-pox grew more mild, and much less frequent;—the other Diseases also less common, but more inflammatory; no malignant Sore-Throats: Many were severely tormented with Coughs, and obstinate asthmatic Disorders.—The Blood now drawn was commonly more dense and viscid than it had been for many Months.

The north-east Wind prevailed at the Begining of *April*, and rendered the Air dry, clear, and pretty cold; the Baroscope high: A showery Season succeeded for four, or five, Days, and then the dry north-east Wind return'd from the 21st it was W.N.W.—The Small-pox still up and down, some of a bad Sort: Many Pleurisies, and Peripneumonies, Rheumatism, Jaundice, and Dropsy frequent; severe Coughs every-where: A vast many are troubled with *Worms*, even Adults, as well as Children.

Though we had some agreeable Weather in *May*, the Summer was wet, cold, and uncomfortable; the Atmosphere thick and foggy, the Barometer seldom high, the S.W. and N.W. Winds were much the most frequent. The Fruits of the Earth did not ripen well, but were watery and insipid; a bad Harvest, bad Grain.—A great Dejection of Spirits, Listlessness, and Lassitude were universally complained of.—The Small-pox became much more numerous in *June*, and were epidemic all the Summer, and rather of a worse Kind than in the Spring, not only here, but every-where in the Neighbourhood; they were frequently confluent, very small, and sometimes black, attended with Hæmorrhages of the Nose, especially in Children; but the Petechiæ were much less common than I expected; sometimes they were very crude, crystalline, and indigested, running into Large Blisters, eroding the Skin greatly.—Rheumatisms, Gout, and

Coughs were in vastly greater Plenty than usual at this Time of the Year.

Now also exactly such a Kind of Fever, as I called, in my *Ist Volume of Epidemics, Febris anginosa*, raged up and down with great Violence, attended with scarlet or pustular Eruptions, and succeeded with great Itching and Desquamation of the Cuticle. In this the Pulse was commonly hard, quick, and small, the Breathing hot, and laborious, with great Oppression on the Præcordia, the Urine sometimes crude and pale, sometimes high-coloured and turbid, but without Sediment; a Delirium generally came on soon.—The Sick commonly bore Bleeding at the Begining with Advantage, and the Blood was often sizy, though much less so in general than in Squinzies of the truly inflammatory Kind; they very seldom however admitted of large Bleeding, scarce indeed of a second.

In all Sorts of Fevers there was a surprizing Disposition to Eruptions of some Kind or other, to Sweats, Soreness of throat and Apthæ.—The Small-pox were more fatal in *August*, and sometimes attended with a very dangerous Ulceration in the Throat, and Difficulty of Swallowing.—Indeed the malignant ulcerous Sore-Throat was now also frequent, probably sometimes complicated with the Small-pox.

The Autumn was much more fair, and comfortable, than the Summer, particularly the Month of *October* was for the greater Part beautiful and serene, the Mercury high; however, the Atmosphere was generally thick, and sometimes very moist, the Wind commonly from the eastern Quarters: *November* was less wet and stormy than usual, and in general warm; the Barometer pretty high, but the Air thick and humid.—At the Begining of *December* the Quicksilver was exceeding high, the Air cold and dry, Wind E.N.E; but from the 6th to the 26th very wet and foggy, sometimes boisterous, and the Barometer sunk very much; towards the End the Easterly Wind returned, raised the Mercury, and restored fine, cold Weather.

During this Period the Small-pox continued epidemic every where, and, though somewhat more mild in *September* and *October*, yet here and there they were very confluent, attended with Spots and Hæmorrhages of the Nose.—In *December* they were often crude, numerous, and undigested to the last, running into very large Vesications, deeply eroding the subjacent Parts: the Crusts of the black confluent many Times remained for at least thirty Days after the Eruption.—The *anginose Fever* also still continued—and we had several of the *malignant Sore-Throats* in *September*, many more in *October*, in *November*, and *December* they were exceeding common in this *Town*, at the *Dock*, and all around us, and carried off a great many Adults, as well as Children.—During this Time likewise catarrhal, mucous Sore-Throats were innumerable, but with little Severity, or Danger.—In *October* particularly, after a few Days of foggy, stormy, rainy Weather, we had from the 12th to the 16th very cold Mornings, and immense hoar Frosts with some Ice, in which Time Hundreds of People were at once seized with a Cough, Sore-Throat, and a great Defluxion from the Nose, Eyes and Mouth, attended with a slight Fever, and more, or less, of a *Rash*, several with great *Fluxes* of the *Belly*.—Coughs, Catarrhs, Rheumatisms and Fluxes were excessively common in *November* and *December*, especially catarrhal Coughs, with which almost every one was in some Degree troubled; and yet there were very few Peripneumonies, or Pleurisies; however, Abundance fell into a pulmonary Phthisis, and many died tabid.

For many Months past we had scarce the slightest Fever, but it was attended with a Sore-Throat, Apthæ, and some Kind of cuticular Eruption, and that too even in pleuritic and peripneumonic Disorders—so greatly did the Constitution of the Air, *&c.* seem disposed to produce Eruptions in all Sorts of feverish Indispositions.—The Blood drawn from the Diseased, during all this Time, hath been very rarely viscid, but generally florid seemingly, especially at the very Begining of the Malady, and of a very loose Texture.

Thus ended the Year 1752.—The following Part of the Winter, and succeeding Spring, was very cold and wet; the cold Weather continued till the Middle of *May*, and made a very backward Spring. Then came on very fine hot Weather, and we had the warmest, and most beautiful Summer, that hath been known for many Years.—The Small-pox, and both catarrhal and malignant Squinzies grew less frequent, and less fatal, from *January* to *May*, when both entirely ceased.—As the Spring advanced, we had several Pleurisies, Peripneumonies, and a vast Number of catarrhal Disorders:—The Blood now drawn was much more dense and viscid in general than had been observed for many Months before.

I have given this short Account of the Constitution of the Air and Diseases, during this Period, in which Sore-Throats of one Kind, or another, were much more frequent than I ever before remember, and with which also cuticular Eruptions of various Sorts were exceedingly common, and this too even in the slightest Fevers that happened.—And this I have particularly done, that perhaps from it some rational Conjectures of the Cause and Nature of such Disorders may be made.—Did the long cold and wet Seasons occasion them, by hindering a due and regular Perspiration? The suppressed Perspirabile grows very acrid, and productive at length of a Variety of Diseases, particularly such as pass under the general Name of Scorbutic, as well as more immediately of Catarrhs, Squinzies, Peripneumonies, Fluxes, Colics, *&c.* which are notoriously the Effects of suppressed Perspiration.—But my present Design is not to enter into Disquisitions of this Nature.—I proceed therefore to give the most exact Account, I possibly can, of the *Malignant, Ulcerous Sore-Throat*, as it raged here during the Period above described, especially in 1752.—To which I shall subjoin the Method of Cure I found most successful.

The *Attack* of this Disease was very different in different Persons.—Sometimes a Rigor, with some Fulness and Soreness of the Throat, and painful Stiffness of the Neck, were the very first Symptoms complained of.—Sometimes alternate Chills and Heats, with some Degree of Head-ach, Giddiness, or Drowsiness, ushered in the Distemper.—It seized others with much more feverish Symptoms, great Pain of the Head, Back, and Limbs, a vast Oppression of the Præcordia, and continual Sighing.—Some grown Persons, on the contrary, moved about for a Day, or two, neither sick or well, as it were, but under Uneasiness and Anxiety till they were obliged to lie for it. Thus various was the Disease at the *Onset*. But it commonly began with Chills and Heats, Load and Pain of the Head, Soreness of Throat and Hoarseness, some Cough, Sickness at Stomach, frequent Vomiting and Purging, in Children especially, which were sometimes very severe; though a contrary State was more common to the Adult.—There was in all a very great Dejection of Spirits, very sudden Weakness, great Heaviness on the Breast, and Faintness, from the very Begining.—The Pulse in general was quick, small and fluttering, though sometimes heavy and undose.—The Urine commonly pale, thin, and crude, however, in many grown Persons in small Quantities, and high-coloured, or like turbid Whey.—The Eyes were heavy, reddish, and as it were weeping,—the Countenance very often full, flushed and bloated, though sometimes pale and sunk.

How slight soever the Disorder might appear in the Day-time, at

Night the Symptoms became greatly aggravated, and the feverish Habit very much encreased, nay, sometimes a Delirium came on the very first Night; and this Exacerbation constantly returned in the Evening through the whole Course of the Disease.—Indeed, when it was considerably on the Decline, I have been often pretty much surprized to find my Patient had passed the whole Night in a Phrenzy, whom I had left tolerably cool and sedate in the Day.

Some few Hours after the Seizure, and sometimes cotemporary with it, a Swelling and Soreness of the Throat was perceived, and the Tonsils became very tumid and inflamed, and many Times the parotid and maxillary Glands swelled very much, and very suddenly, even at the very Begining, sometimes so much as even to threaten Strangulation. The Fauces also very soon appeared of a high florid Red, or rather of a bright Crimson Colour, very shining and glossy; and most commonly on the *Uvula, Tonsils, Velum Palatinum*, and back Part of the *Pharynx*, several whitish, or Ash-coloured Spots appeared scattered up and down, which oftentimes encreased very fast, and soon covered one, or both the Tonsils, Uvula, *&c*: these in Event proved the *Sloughs* of superficial Ulcers (which sometimes however eat very deep into the Parts.) The Tongue at this Time, though only white and moist at the Top, was very foul at the Root, and covered with a thick yellowish, or brown Coat.—The Breath also now began to be very nauseous, which offensive Smell encreased hourly, and in some became at length intolerable, and that too sometimes even to the Patients themselves.

The second, or third Day, every Symptom became much more aggravated, and the Fever much more considerable, and those, that had struggled with it tolerably well for thirty or forty Hours, were forced to submit.—The Restlessness and Anxiety greatly encreased, as well as the Difficulty in Swallowing.—The Head was very giddy, pained, and loaded; there was generally more or less of a Delirium, sometimes a Pervigilium and perpetual Phrenzy, though others lay very stupid, but often starting and muttering to themselves.—The Skin was very hot, dry and rough; there was very rarely any Disposition to sweat. The Urine pale, thin, crude, often yellowish, and turbid. Sometimes a Vomiting was urgent, and sometimes a very great Looseness, in Children particularly. The Sloughs were now much enlarged, and of a darker Colour, and the surrounding Parts tended much more to a livid Hue.—The Breathing became much more difficult, with a Kind of a *rattling Stertor*, as if the

Patient was actually strangling, the Voice being exceeding hoarse and hollow, exactly resembling that from *venereal Ulcers in the Fauces*; this Noise in Speaking and Breathing was so peculiar, that any Person in the least conversant with the Disease might easily know it by this odd Noise; from whence indeed the *Spanish Physicians* gave it the Name of *Garotillo*, expressing the Noise such make as are strangling with a Rope.—I never observed in one of them the shrill, barking Noise, that we frequently hear in inflammatory Squinzies. The Breath of all the Diseased was very nauseous, of some insufferably foetid, especially in the Advance of the Distemper to a Crisis; and many about the fourth or fifth Day spit off a vast Quantity of stinking, purulent Mucus, tinged sometimes with Blood, and sometimes the Matter was quite livid, and of an abominable Smell. The Nostrils likewise in many were greatly inflamed and excoriated, continually dripping down a most sharp *Ichor*, or *sanious Matter*, so excessively acrid, that it not only corroded the Lips, Cheeks, and Hands of the Children, that laboured under the Disease, but even the Fingers and Arms of the very Nurses, that attended them: As this Ulceration of the Nostrils came on, it commonly caused an almost incessant Sneezing in the Children, but few Adults were affected with it, at least to any considerable Degree. It was surprizing what Quantities of Matter some Children discharged this Way, which they would often rub on their Face, Hands and Arms, and blister them all over.—A sudden Stoppage of this Rheum from the Mouth and Nostrils actually choaked several Children; and some swallowed such Quantities of it, as occasioned Excoriations of the Intestines, violent Gripings, Dysentery, *&c*; nay, even Excoriations of the Anus and Buttocks.—Not only the Nostrils, Fauces, *&c.* were greatly affected by this extreamly sharp Matter, but the Wind-pipe itself was sometimes much corroded by it, and Pieces of its internal Membrane were spit up, with much Blood and Corruption, and the Patients lingered on for a considerable Time, and at length died tabid; tho' there were more frequent Instances of its falling more suddenly and violently on the Lungs, and killing in a peripneumonic Manner.

I was astonished sometimes to see several swallow with tolerable Ease, though the Tumour of the Tonsils and Throat, the Quantity of thick Mucus, and the rattling Noise in breathing, were very terrible; which I think pretty clearly shews, that this malignant Squinzey was more from the Acrimony and Abundance of the Humors than the Violence of the Inflammation.

Most commonly the *Angina* came on before the *Exanthemata*, but many Times the cuticular Eruption appeared before the Sore-Throat, and was sometimes very considerable, though there was little, or no Pain in the Fauces; on the contrary, a very severe Angina seized some Patients, that had no Manner of Eruption, and yet, even in these Cases, a very great Itching and Desquamation of the Skin sometimes ensued, but this was chiefly in grown Persons, very rarely in Children.—In general, however, a very considerable *Efflorescence* broke out on the Surface of the Body, particularly in Children, and it most commonly happened the second, third, or fourth Day; sometimes it was partial, sometimes it covered almost the whole Body, tho' very seldom on the Face: Sometimes it was of an *Erysipelatous* Kind, sometimes more *pustular*; the Pustules were frequently very eminent, and of a deep, fiery, red Colour, particularly on the Breast and Arms, but oftentimes they were very small, and might be better felt than seen, and gave a very odd Kind of Roughness to the Skin. The Colour of the Efflorescence was commonly of a crimson Hue, or as if the Skin had been smeared over with *Juice of Rasberries*, and this even to the Fingers Ends; and the Skin appeared inflamed and swoln as it were, the Arms, Hands and Fingers were often evidently so, and very stiff, and somewhat painful.—This crimson Colour of the Skin seemed indeed peculiar to this Disease.—Though the Eruption seldom failed of giving some manifest Relief to the Patient, as to Anxiety, Sickness at Stomach, Vomiting, Purging, *&c.* yet I observed an universal, fiery Eruption on some Persons, without the least Abatement of the Symptoms, nay, almost every Symptom seemed more aggravated, particularly the Fever, Load at Breast, Anxiety, Delirium; and I knew more than one, or two Patients die in the most raging Phrenzy, covered with the most universal, fiery Rash, I ever saw: So that, as in the highly confluent Small-pox, it seemed only to denote the *Quantity of the Disease*, as I may term it.

I had under my Care a young Gentleman, about twelve Years of Age, whose Tongue, Fauces, and Tonsils were as black as Ink, and he swallowed with extream Difficulty; he continually spit off immense Quantities of a black, sanious, and very foetid Matter for at least eight or ten Days—about the seventh Day, his Fever being somewhat abated, he fell into a bloody Dysentery, tho' the bloody, sanious, foetid Expectoration still continued with a most violent Cough.—He at length indeed got over it, to the very great Surprize of every one that saw him.—Now in this Patient, as severe and universal a *Rash* broke out upon him the second and third Day, as I ever met with, and the Itching of his Skin was so intolerable, that he tore it all over his Body in a most shocking Manner; yet this very great and timely Eruption very little relieved his Fever and Phrenzy, or prevented the other dreadful Symptoms mentioned.

An early and kindly Eruption, however, was most commonly a very good Omen, and, when succeeded by a very copious Desquamation of the Cuticle, one of the most favourable Symptoms that occurred; but when the Eruption turned of a dusky or livid Colour, or prematurely or suddenly receded, every Symptom grew worse, and the utmost Danger impended, especially if purple, or black, Spots appeared up and down, as sometimes happened; the Urine grew limpid, and Convulsions came on, or a fatal Suffocation soon closed the Tragedy.

The Disease was generally at the Height about the *fifth* or *sixth* Day in young Persons, in the elder not so soon, and the *Crisis* many Times was not till the *eleventh* or *twelfth*, and then very imperfect: Some Adults however were carried off in two or three Days, the Distemper either falling on the Lungs, and killing in a peripneumonic Manner, or on the Brain, and the Patient either died raving, or comatose.—In some the Disease brought on a very troublesome Cough, purulent Expectoration, Hæmoptoë and Hectic, in which they lingered on for several Weeks, and then died tabid.

If a gentle easy Sweat came on the third or fourth Day, if the Pulse became more slow, firm, and equal; if the Sloughs of the Fauces cast off in a kindly Manner, and appeared at the Bottom tolerably clean and florid; if the Breathing was more soft and free, and some Degree of Vigour and Quickness returned in the Eyes, all was well, and a salutary Crisis followed soon by a Continuance of the Sweat, and a turbid, subsiding, farinaceous Urine, a plentiful Expectoration, and a very large Desquamation of the Cuticle.—But if a Rigor came on, and the Exanthemata suddenly disappeared, or turned livid; if the Pulse grew very small and quick, and the Skin remained hot and parched as it were, the Breathing more difficult, the Eyes dead and glassy, the Urine pale and limpid, a Phrenzy or Coma succeeded, with a coldish, clammy Sweat on the Face, or Extremities, Life was despaired of, especially if a *Singultus* and *Choaking,* or *Gulphing* in the Throat, attended, with sudden, liquid, involuntary, livid Stools, intolerably foetid.—In some few Patients I observed, some Time before the fatal Period, not only the Face bloated, sallow, shining, and greasy as it were, but the whole Neck vastly swoln, and of a cadaverous Look; and even the whole Body became, in some Degree, œdematous, and the Impression of a Finger would remain fixed in a Part, the Skin not rising again as usual; an Indication, that the Blood stagnated in the Capillaries, and that the Elasticity of the Fibres was quite lost.

As there were so many different Kinds of Squinzies and eruptive Disorders, during the Period, in which the malignant ulcerous Sore-Throat raged, the Likeness of the Symptoms, at the very Begining of these various Diseases, made it not a little difficult, to the younger and less experienced Practitioners especially, to know what Methods to pursue at the *Onset*; particularly as to the common Evacuations; seeing it was now certain, from sufficient Experience, that in what is called the *malignant, ulcerous Sore-Throat,* Bleeding and Purging, to any Degree at least, were utterly improper.

Tho' I really think our *Gentlemen in the Medical Way*, that practise in this Part of the Kingdom, are in general as careful, capable, and judicious as in most Parts of *England*, yet I took some Pains with them to make them comprehend the Nature of this singular and uncommon Distemper, and to distinguish it aright from some other reigning Disorders, that bore no small Resemblance to it.—And having desired them to attend to the small, quick, unequal fluttering Pulse at the Attack of this malignant Squinzey, though indeed it was sometimes full and undose, but even then heavy and unequal—to the sudden great Dejection of Spirits and Strength—perpetual Anxiety, Sighing, and great Oppression on the Præcordia—heavy, dull, watery, and as it were weeping Eye—pale, crude, thin Urine, though often turbid, like Whey—to the whitish, but commonly moist Tongue, though considerably furred near the Root—to the shining, crimson Colour of the Fauces, with interspersed white, or ash-coloured Spots or Blotches, with a nauseous and sometimes very foetid Breath—to the scarlet or crimson Efflorescence (in some erysipelatous, in others pustular) on the Hands, Arms, Neck, Breast, *&c.*—Symptoms that attended this Disease, even on the very first Days; they distinguished better, proceeded with more Caution, and with greater Success.—I met with too many Instances before, of rash, large Bleeding and Purging in this Distemper, nay, some were weak enough to tell me the Blood, they had drawn, was very *fine* and *rich*; *florid* truly I found it as *Lamb*'s *Blood,* but so soft and loose that you might cut it with a Feather, giving off little or no *Serum*, but having exactly such an Appearance as when *Spirit of Harts-horn* is poured to the Blood, just as it runs from the Vein, which prevents its natural Coagulation.

I will not say but that, in some plethoric adult Persons, some Blood may be drawn at the very Begining of this Disease, and I have in some few ordered it with Advantage, particularly as to the *anginose Symptoms*, and where the Difficulty of Breathing also was considerable; but I must say, a Repetition of the Bleeding to any considerable Degree is extreamly detrimental, where the first Blood especially was of such a loose and soft Texture; for the second or third will be always found a *mere sanious Gore*, as I have too often noted—nay, sometimes I have observed the first Blood drawn covered with a very *thin, whitish*, or *Lead-coloured Skin*, pretty tenacious; but immediately underneath it was a *greenish, soft Kind of Jelly*, and at Bottom a very loose, *black Crassamentum*, scarce at all cohering.—This Appearance of the Blood, however, as much forbids further Bleeding as that above described, and is mostly observed when there is a throbbing Pulse, and great Heat at the Access of the Distemper.—I profess I was myself not a little mistaken in two or three Cases at the first breaking out of this Fever; one of them I took for a true Peripneumony, but the Sore-Throat, Scarlet Eruption, Stench of the Breath, and even Petechiæ very soon coming on, too plainly convinced me what was in Truth the Disease.

I have very often met with this buffy, or sizy, Appearance of the Blood in the Begining of Malignant Fevers, and yet Blood, drawn two or three Days after from the very same Persons, hath been quite loose, dissolved and sanious as it were.—Too many Instances of this very lately occurred to me amongst the *French Captives here*, who died by *Dozens* of a *contagious, pestilential Fever*, very frequently attended with Petechiæ, and a bloody Dysentery.—In this Fever (as well as all others) the *French Surgeons* bled of Course every Day, or at least every other Day.—And I several Times saw the Blood of some of the *Officers* (thus treated) a mere *sanious Gore* on the third or fourth Bleeding, though considerably sizy at the first.—And yet so preposterous was their Practice, that, at the same Time they were so busy with the *Lancet*, they *gorged their Patients with the strongest Bouillon, that Beef, Mutton, &c. could make*, and this too though they were in a constant Delirium, were covered with black or purple Spots, and had their Tongues as black as Ink, and as dry and rough as a Pumice-stone.—I am very certain great Numbers fell a Sacrifice to this absurd Practice.

This buffy Appearance of the Blood, at the very Begining of contagious, pestilential Fevers, doth not invalidate what I have said, in my *Essay on Fevers*, of the Effect of *contagious Effluvia* on the Blood in such Fevers, but rather confirms it:—for though they tend to dissolve, and actually at length do destroy the *Crasis* of the Blood, yet Persons, of a very viscid, dense State of Blood, may be seized with a contagious, malignant Fever, and the Blood may appear very sizy and buffy on Bleeding at the very *Attack*, but, notwithstanding this, the Action of the *contagious Ferment* (if I may be allowed the Expression) will more and more dissolve the Blood, and at last render it a mere *sanious Putrilage*, and so it will appear on subsequent Bleedings.—And therefore, where there is just Reason to fear a contagious Malignity in a Fever, we should proceed with the utmost Caution as to repeated Bleeding, especially as it will be constantly found, that the Pulse, as well as the Strength, sink vastly after the second or third Bleeding, and truly sometimes very surprizingly after the first.

But to return to my Subject.—Whenever I was called to Persons seized with this Malady, at the very Begining, I generally, instead of Bleeding, ordered a Clyster of Milk, Sugar, and Salt to be injected to unload the Intestines, especially if the Patient was costive.—But, when a Purging attends the Attack, a few Grains of *torrefied Rhubarb* with *Species e Scordio, Decoct. alb.* &c. are proper; and if the Diarrhœa is profuse, a Spoonful or two of *Decoct. Fracastorii Fulleri* may be frequently given, which is, in such Cases, a very efficacious Medicine.—If Nausea and Vomiting were urgent, I ordered a gentle *Emetic*, especially for Adults, which was so far from aggravàting the Pain of the Throat, as might be imagined, that it generally greatly relieved it—nay, in Children it was often necessary to make them puke frequently with a little *Oxymel. Scillit. Essence of Antimony*, or the like, otherwise the vast Amass of tenacious Mucus would quite choak them.

I then immediately put the Patient on a *saline Mixture of Salt of Wormwood*, or *volatile Salt of Harts-horn*, and *Juice of Lemon* with *Aq. Alexeter. Simpl.* to which was added *Pulv. Contrayerv. C.* with a small Quantity of *Myrrh* and *Saffron*; or these last were given in a *Bolus*, with a few Grains of *Nitre*, if the Fever ran pretty high—the Addition also of a Grain or two of *Camphire* was very useful for the Adult, where the Stomach would bear it; when it would not, I used *Julep è Camphor.* or *Acetum Camphoratum* with *Syrup* of *black Currants*, Rasberries, or the like.—The second or third Day, to the saline Mixture, or a temperate Cordial Julep, I added some of my *Tinct. Cort. Peruvian. Alexipharmac.* which, at this Time of the Disease, I found greatly preferable to the *Bark* in Substance; as it much more tends to promote the Eruption of the Exanthemata, and doth not by far so much hinder the Coming on of Sweats, which at all Times of this Distemper are of the highest Service, provided they are gentle, uniform, and universal.—Indeed it was with great Difficulty the Sick could be brought to sweat at all, but whenever moderate, equally diffused Sweats came on the third, fourth, or fifth Day, or even later, they were critical and salutary, the Urine grew immediately more concocted, and forthwith deposited a very large Quantity of *Clay-coloured*, or *pale lateritious Sediment*, though before crude, thin, or limpid; and therefore I always endeavoured to promote them by soft, easy Diaphoretics, and plentiful Dilution with Barely-water, thin Whey, Gruel, Tea or the like.—I do not remember I had one Patient miscarry, who fell into soft, easy, universal Sweats, tho' the Itching, that sometimes came on with them, was almost intolerable, but generally the Sweat soon abated the Itching; at least it constantly lessened the Fever; and the Purging (if there was any) immediately ceased; the Tumour of the Neck, Parotids, *&c.* subsided greatly also on the Appearance of a kindly plentiful Diaphoresis: The Sweats were commonly very rank and foetid, and that even in Children.

I commonly gave *Elixir Vitrioli* with the *Tincture* of the *Bark*, (except to very young Children, which is an excellent *anti-putrescent Alexipharmac*; and I frequently ordered the *Elixir* to be taken out of an *Infusion of a roasted Seville-orange* in *Claret* or *red Port-Wine and Water*, which is a very pleasant and not an ineffectual Composition.

There was an absolute Necessity of washing out the Mouth and Fauces very frequently—the *Gargle*, I commonly ordered, was a *Decoction of Figs, red Rose-leaves, Myrrh* and *Honey* in *rough Cyder*, and a thin *Mucilage* of *Quinceseeds* with Syrup of Rasberries, or black Currants; and a little *Tincture of Myrrh, per se*, and *Spirit of Vitriol*, was to be taken by Spoonfuls every now and then, especially after *Gargling.*—And I also directed the *Fumes* of *red Rose-leaves, Chamomile-flowers, Myrrh*, and *Camphire*, boiled in *Vinegar*, to be drawn in with the Breath very often, as hot as the Patients could well bear it, which gave very great and speedy Relief.

Though the Swelling of the Neck, parotid Glands, *&c.* would sometimes come on so sudden, great and violent, as to endanger a Suffocation, yet in general I took this external Tumour to be partly critical, and therefore endeavoured to promote it by *acrid Cataplasms, Blisters,* &c. nay I have several Times blistered the Throat from Ear to Ear with great Success.—These Applications are useful in common Squinzeys; much more so in this, where the Humours were so exceeding sharp and malignant.

As there was frequently a very great Tension and Tumour of the Belly, and at the same Time also some Degree of a Suppression of Urine, an *emollient Fotus* with some of the *Carminative Seeds,* or a few *Chamomile-flowers* boiled in *Milk* and *Water,* and a Clyster of the same with *salt* and *Sugar,* were necessary to promote the Discharge of Stool, Wind and Urine, which gave immediate Ease to the Bowels, and withal greatly facilitated the Respiration, by giving a more *free Play* to the *Diaphragm.*—Indeed if the Abdomen was very tense, and the Patient costive, about the fifth, or sixth Day, I generally gave a *Dose* of *Rhubarb, Manna,* or *lenitive Electuary*— and after that commonly the *Bark* in *Substance*; but I never so ordered it when the Belly was very tumid and constipated, nor until some Signs of *Coction,* or a begining *Desquamation* of the *Cuticle* appeared; for I found my *Tincture,* or a *Decoction of the Bark,* answer full as well, nay better, as causing much less Oppression on the Breast.—I now also used a *Kind of Resin of the Bark,* made with *Spirit of Wine,* which I much prefer to the common Extract, as it sits much lighter on the Stomach, and keeps much better; and therefore I think is more proper for an *officinal Medicine.*

However improper Purging might be at the Begining of this Distemper, gentle, easy *Cathartics,* as *Rhubarb, Manna,* &c. were necessary at the End to carry off the putrid Colluvies of the Intestines, which otherwise protracted the feverish Heats, and occasioned great Weakness, Want of Appetite, timid Bellies, and great Obstructions of the Glands; nay I was often obliged to give repeated Doses of *Calomel* to carry off the Swellings of the parotid and maxillary Glands, which otherwise frequently remained a long Time much swoln and indurated, and, at length, sometimes suppurated:—Indeed I several Times found it necessary to rub them with a *Mercurial Unguent* before I could dissolve the Tumors; *Calomel* was also further useful in destroying the *Worms,* with which a vast Number were at this Time especially troubled.—But in general after a Purge, or two, the Sick soon recovered a keen Appetite, Strength and Spirits: Many however required frequent Purging, a Continuance of the *Bark*, *Æthiops mineral*, &c. for a considerable Time, and then a Course of Asses-milk, and an open Country-Air to prevent a wasting Hectic; of which some died eight, or ten, Weeks, after the Disease first seized them.

This was undoubtedly a *Fever* of the *malignant, pestilential Kind*, in which the Blood became highly acrimonious, dissolved, and putrescent. That it was very greatly contagious no one doubts, as it very often infected whole Families, especially the younger Persons.—And that this Contagion generated a very great Degree of Acrimony in the Blood is most evident from the History of the Disease.—I have elsewhere noted that Contagion acts in the Blood as Acrimony: Perhaps the *contagious Miasmata* are only the highly exalted *Salino-sulphureous* Particles and Vapours that exhale from the diseased infecting Body.—It is well known the Stench of putrid Carcasses, gangrened Limbs, the polluted, stinking Air of Jails, *&c.* destroy the *Crasis* of the Blood, and bring on malignant, pestilential Fevers; just as the putrid Sanies of a gangrened Limb, absorbed into the Blood, brings on a Fever of the same Kind.—It is certain the *pestilential Effluvia* in the true Plague bring on the most healthy, in a very few Hours, a putrid Dissolution and gangrenous Disposition of the Blood—and truly this malignant Sore-Throat was in some Cases found very little inferior to it in Virulence, not only the Fauces, but the Lungs, Intestines, *&c.* having appeared gangrenous on Dissections, and the whole Mass of Blood turned into a putrid Gore.—That an exceeding small Quantity of morbid Matter will infect the whole Mass of Blood is most certain from the Experiment of inoculating the Small-pox, in which it is found, that very much less than a Grain of the variolous Matter is fully sufficient to bring on that Distemper; nor is that surprizing when we too well know what dreadful Effects arise from the minutest Quantity imaginable of the Virus of a Viper, or mad Dog.

Though this malignant ulcerous Squinzey seemed to be a *Disease sui Generis*, yet it certainly had a very great Resemblance of the *Febris anginosa*, which I formerly described in my *first Volume de Aëre & Morbis Epidemicis*; and it is pretty remarkable, that such a Kind of Fever now also greatly prevailed up and down this Part of the Country; but indeed the anginose Fever had very much more of an inflammatory Nature than the malignant Sore-Throat now treated of, and the Blood was commonly found much more dense and viscid in the former than in the latter, and of Course would much better admit of Bleeding.—But in Truth it may be in this, as in many other epidemic Disorders, particularly the Small-pox, Measles, Scarlet Fever, *&c.*—the general Disease is greatly diversified by the particular Constitution of the Patients.—Thus the variolous Contagion in one of strong elastic Fibres, and a very viscid dense Blood, brings on a very high inflammatory Fever,—in another of weak, lax Fibres, and a loose dissolved Blood, a low, putrid, nervous Fever, not sufficient to protrude the Pustules in a kindly Manner, much less to bring them to a laudable Maturation.—In a Word, the high inflammatory Small-pox differ as much, or more, from the low malignant Kind, as the *Febris anginosa* from the *pestilential ulcerous Sore-Throat.*—How greatly doth the Scarlet Fever, described by *Morton*, differ from that mentioned by *Sydenham*?—And indeed, although the same specific Contagion always produces the same specific Disease, yet it greatly differs in different Persons, and is to be treated accordingly.—There were certainly some of these ulcerous Sore-Throats with a pretty smart Fever, that bore Bleeding at the Begining with Advantage, and a much cooler Regimen was necessary in some than in others,—nay I was obliged in several Cases to give Nitre with the Diaphoretics.—But I must confess, in general, much warmer Medicines were necessary in this than in most other Fevers; and that too sometimes when the Heat was very considerable, otherwise the Pulse would sink surprizingly, and an astonishing Anxiety, and Oppression, immediately succeeded. —I have really been obliged to give such warm *Alexipharmacs* in this Distemper (and that too many Times to very young Persons) as nothing but repeated Experience could have induced me to order; as *Saffron, Camphire, Pulv. Contrayerv. Confect. Cardiac. Theriac. Andromach*, warm Cyder, mulled Wine and Water, *Tinct. Cortic. Alexipharmac.* &c. and this with a Success that was well known, and justified the Practice.

The Word *Fever*, as promiscuously used in the Practice of Physic, is not a little vague and undetermined.—There are some Disorders, that pass under that general Name, which are best cured even by raising the Fever, to instance only in some Quartan Agues and low, nervous Fevers.—And the malignant Squinzey, here described, is another Species of Fever, which evidently proves that all acute Diseases are not to be treated merely with Evacuations, and cooling Medicines—proper Dilution is unquestionably useful in all

Fevers, but certainly some require more than *Barley-water* and *Limonade.*—But I have already said several Things on this Head in my *Essay on Fevers*; and shall at present only add a Word or two on the Use of *volatile alcalious Salts* in Fevers of the putrid pestilential, or petechial Kind; in which I fear they are too often very improperly administered.

And here I must observe, that, in all Fevers of this Nature, the Blood is always found too much broken and dissolved, and at length becomes highly acrimonious, and as it were sanious and putrid. Whatever therefore tends to promote the Acrimony and Dissolution of the Blood must be very apt to bring on such Fevers, and encrease their Malignity, when they happen; but volatile alcalious Salts do both in an eminent Degree; for though they may retard the Putrefaction of the Flesh of Animals, and even in some Measure of the Blood, out of the Body (and so will *Arsenic*, or *Sublimate-corrosive*) yet mixed with the Blood, whilst actually under the Power of Circulation and the *Vis Vitæ*, they certainly hasten its Dissolution, and consequent Putrefaction; even mixed with the Blood out of the Body, or rather as it runs from the Vein, they quite destroy the Texture of the Blood-globules, nearly in the same Manner as the Poison of a Viper by dissolving the *Copula*, or Cohæsion of the component Particles; and the Blood of the most Robust (nay even the most buffy Blood of Horses, as I have often tried) thus managed never concretes, as usual, into a solid *Crassamentum*, and throws off its *Serum*, but remains ever after a loose, dissolved Gore, or Sanies.—Now let me farther observe, that when these volatile alcalious Salts (or Spirits) are taken in large Quantities, and frequently, even by Persons in Health, they are well known to bring on feverish Heats, Hæmorrhages, spongy bleeding Gums, stinking Breath, rank Urine, *&c.* Symptoms that sufficiently indicate a begining Dissolution, and Putridity of the Blood.

Moreover these broken, dissolved Blood-globules are very apt to enter into the serous and lymphatic Arteries, and there, not finding a free Passage through their Ramifications, stagnate and corrupt, and at length even corrode these exceeding tender Vessels, particularly when saturated with acrimonious Salts, which at the same Time also greatly irritate these very minute Canals, encrease the Heat, and so cause a more speedy Corruption both of the Humours and Vessels; and when the putrid *Lymph* and *Serum* is absorbed into the Mass of Blood, it greatly hastens the general Corruption.

Volatile alcalious Salts, even applied externally to the Skin, very speedily corrode and ulcerate, and it is certainly Fact, that given internally they heat vastly more, Quantity for Quantity, than the warmest *vegetable Alexipharmacks.*—And that, I think, not so much by encreasing the projectile Force, and Circulation, of the Blood, as by causing an intestine Motion and Effervescence in it; for, by the most accurate Experiments, it is found that Solutions of the volatile alcaline Salts weaken the Tone of the Fibres, and Power of the Vessels, and consequently the *Momentum of the Blood* in the regular Course of Circulation.—And we eventually find, that, when the Blood abounds with very acrid Salts, the Pulse becomes weak, small, quick and fluttering, as in the highly scorbutic, and that corrupt, acrimonious State of Blood, which brings on the putrid Fever, antecedent to some Mortifications *ab internâ Causâ*, as they call it; in both which the Powers of Nature sink greatly, and particularly the Strength of the arterial Vibrations, tho' they may encrease in Quickness, to compensate for the Want of that natural Vigour, and Fulness, which is observed in a free and firm Pulsation of an Artery duly filled with Blood, and properly actuated.—The extraordinary Bigness and Flaccidity of the Heart, that is commonly noted in scorbutic and pestilential Cases, are owing to the Weakness and great Relaxation of its muscular Fibres.—That peculiar Kind of biting Heat, that we commonly feel on the Skin of Persons labouring under putrid, malignant Fevers, seems to arise from the Abundance of acrid Salts and Sulphurs in the Blood, and its intestine Motion, and not from its increased projectile Force; for, on first touching the Skin, the Heat seems very little, if at all, above the natural, but, by continuing the Finger a longer Time on it, you are sensible of a disagreeable Scalding in it, which Sensation even remains in the Finger for some small Time after you have quite removed it from the sick Person: This *Doctor Pringle* hath judiciously noted in his excellent *Treatise on the Diseases of the Army*; and *Galen*, as he candidly observes, long before him.—This *Monsieur Quesnoy* calls *la Chaleur d'Acrimonie*, and very justly distinguishes it from *la Chaleur d' Inflammation.*—The Sensation, in Truth, is as different as touching a very hot Piece of dry Wood, and dipping your Finger into tepid Spirit of Hartshorn.—And I think this observation evidently proves the Abundance of acrimonious Salts thrown off by Perspiration in these very putrid Fevers. That peculiar burning Heat also, which the Sick often feel within, in such

Diseases, though the external Parts of the Body are actually cold, probably arises from the same Cause.—And I cannot but think the Heat, observable in Fevers, preceding and attending Mortifications *ab internâ Causâ*, is generated by the Acrimony and intestine Motion of the Humours; not certainly from a rapid projectile Motion, for the Pulse is then always found weak and small, though quick. The surprizingly speedy and great Stench, Swelling, and sanious Hæmorrhages from all the Outlets of the Bodies of such as die in putrid, malignant Fevers, are Arguments of the great intestine Motion, Rarefaction, and Acrimony of the Humors.—This was the Case commonly of those that died of the malignant, anginose Fever above described. I have known the whole Body swell vastly, even to the Ends of the Fingers and Toes, with a cadaverous Lividity, though almost quite cold, and an intolerable Stench even before the Person was actually dead, Blood issuing, at the same Time, from the Ears, Nose, Mouth, and Guts; and this too where the Pulse had been very weak and small, tho' exceeding quick, from the very Beginning.—Was not this, from much Air, generated in the Blood by the intestine Motion, Heat, and Putridity, which are well known to generate Air? Is not the Emphysema, observable in some Sphacelations, from the same Cause?

But to proceed, if we consider the Generation and Nature of animal Salts, perhaps we shall see a little further into this Matter.—The strongest vegetable Acids, we take in with our Food, are by the *Vis Vitæ* soon changed into a *neutral*, or a Kind of *ammoniacal Salts*, and by being longer and longer exposed to the Action of the Vessels, and Heat of the Blood, they more and more approach to an alcaline Nature, and at length would become actually alcaline, were they not diluted, washed off, and corrected by acescent Drink and Diet.—A Person that lives on nothing but mere Water, and Flesh or Fish, without any Thing either acid or acescent, soon contracts a very great Rankness in all his Humours; he grows feverish, and at length his Blood runs into a State of Putrefaction.—The Blood of those that die of Famine becomes highly acrimonious, which begets Fever, Phrenzy, and such a Degree of Putrefaction, as is utterly destructive of the vital Principles. A very melancholy Instance of which I once met with in a poor Gentleman, who obstinately starved himself to Death, and would not, for many Days, either by Force or Persuasion, swallow any Kind of Food, or a Drop of Liquor.—He soon grew feverish, flushed in his Face, and very hot in his Head; his

Pulse was Small, but very quick; in four or five Days his Breath became exceedingly offensive, his Lips, dry, black, parched, his Teeth and Mouth foul, black, bloody, his Urine (when it could be saved) vastly high coloured, and stinking, as much as if it had been kept a Month; at length he trembled continually, could not stand, much less walk, raved and dozed alternately, fell into convulsive Agonies frequently, in which he sometimes sweated pretty much about the Head and Breast, though his Extremities were quite cold, pale, and shrivelled; the Sweat was of a very dark yellow Colour, and of a most nauseous Stench.

It is certain also, that, if the animal Salts are not duly and constantly carried off by Urine, they are highly destructive, as in *Ischuries*, for they continually advance more and more to an alcaline State.—It is not so much from an encreased Quantity, as the Acrimony of the Juices, that an obstinate Suppression of Urine becomes fatal; for I have known it very soon so, where the Patient hath had very large Discharges by Sweat and Stool during the whole Time of the Suppression; particularly I remember, many Years ago, a *renal Ischury* fatal to a corpulent Lady the eleventh Day from the Stoppage, though she was twice bled very largely, and kept purging the whole Time, and consequently did not die from a Redundance of Humours.—She made not a Drop of Urine from the Time of her Seizure to her Death, though she took very largely of *Cantharides* in Substance and Tincture, as well as many other Medicines, particularly large Doses of *Calomel.* Indeed, although I have frequently known *Cantharides* given with very good Effect in *Ischuries*, yet, if they do not answer speedily, but are long continued in large Quantities, I fear they co-operate with the acrid Salts, and hasten the Death of the Patient, by bringing on a Delirium and Convulsions, as I have had the Misfortune to see more than once.

But to the Point in Hand.—The Formation of volatile alcaline Salts in the Body seems not much unlike the Production of them out of the Body.—Let any Kind of green Plant, even the most acid, be pressed together in a large Heap, it soon begins to heat, and gradually grows more and more hot (to such an intense Degree at length, if the Quantity be very large, as to break out into an actual Flame) and this Effervescence soon turns the whole Mass putrid, and the acid and essential Salts of the Plant into volatile Alcalies, which may be distilled from the putrid Mass, and are in no Respect essentially different from the volatile alcaly Salts raised from animal

Substances; both the one and the other are ultimately the Effects of Heat and Motion on the Salts of Vegetables, and the longer, and stronger, these are acted upon by the Force and Heat of our Solids and Fluids, so much the more are they exalted to an alcaline State, in which they are absolutely unfit for the common Uses of Life; nay, exceedingly destructive, if they greatly abound, as in very putrid, pestilential, and petechial Fevers they unquestionably do; and therefore, I think, in such Cases, the Exhibition of volatile alcalious Salts to the sick is adding Fewel to the Fire, for they certainly dissolve or break the Globules of the Blood, and thence more speedily bring on a general Putrefaction.—These Salts, even applied externally to the Skin, soon excite a gangrænous Ulcer; and, when the Blood is largely stocked with them, it becomes a Kind of fiery Lixivium, which is greatly destructive of the *nervous Fibrillæ*, and *ultima Vascula.*—And this indeed would be more certainly, frequently, and speedily the Case than it is, if the plentiful Use of Acids, Diluents, and soft mucilaginous Things, in Drink and Diet, did not prevent it, by washing off and correcting them; as we see Juice of Lemon and Vinegar quite take off their Acrimony; indeed thus managed they are, in many Diseases, turned into very useful Medicines.

Before I conclude, I beg Leave to insert the following extraordinary Case, as it is not altogether foreign to the Purpose.

I had lately under my Care a Gentleman of Fortune and Family, who so habituated himself to the Use of vast Quantities of the *volatile Salts*, that Ladies commonly smell to, that at length he would eat them in a very astonishing Manner, as other People eat *sugared Carraway Seeds.*—A Δριμυφαγεία with a Vengeance!—The Consequence soon was, that he brought on a hectic Fever, vast Hæmorrhages from the Intestines, Nose, and Gums, every one of his Teeth dropped out, and he could eat nothing solid; he wasted vastly in his Flesh, and his Muscles became as soft and flabby as those of a new-born Infant; and broke out all over his Body in Pustules, which itched most intolerably, so that he scratched himself continually, and tore his Skin with his Nails in a very shocking Manner; his Urine was always excessively high coloured, turbid, and very foetid.—He was at last, with great Difficulty, persuaded to leave this pernicious Custom, but he had so effectually ruined his Constitution, that, though he rubbed on in a very miserable Manner for several Months, he died tabid, and in the highest Degree of a

Marasmus;—and I am persuaded, he would have died much sooner, had he not constantly drank very freely of the most fine and generous Wines, and daily used large Quantities of Asses-milk, and anti-scorbutic Juices well acidulated with Juice of Seville-oranges, Lemons, *&c.*

But, after all, I am so far from thinking the *volatile Alcaly-salts* should be struck out of the *Materia Medica*, and condemning their Use in all Cases, that I am very certain they may be given with great Advantage in very many.—But, in Truth, I still except those above-mentioned.

INDEX I.

Of SUBJECTS.

A.

C.

D.

E.

F.

I.

K.

L.

M.

N.

O.

P.

Q.

R.

S.

T.

V.

INDEX II.

Of AUTHORS.

A.

B.

C.

D.

E.

F.

G.

H.

J.

L.

M.

W.

INDEX

To the Dissertation on the Malignant, Ulcerous Sore-Throat.

A.

B.

C.

D.

E.

F.

G.

H.

I.

L.

M.

N.

O.

P.

U. V.

W.